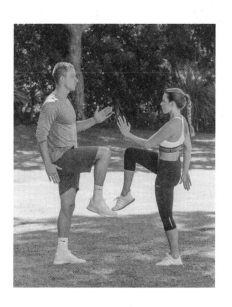

the *buddy* workout

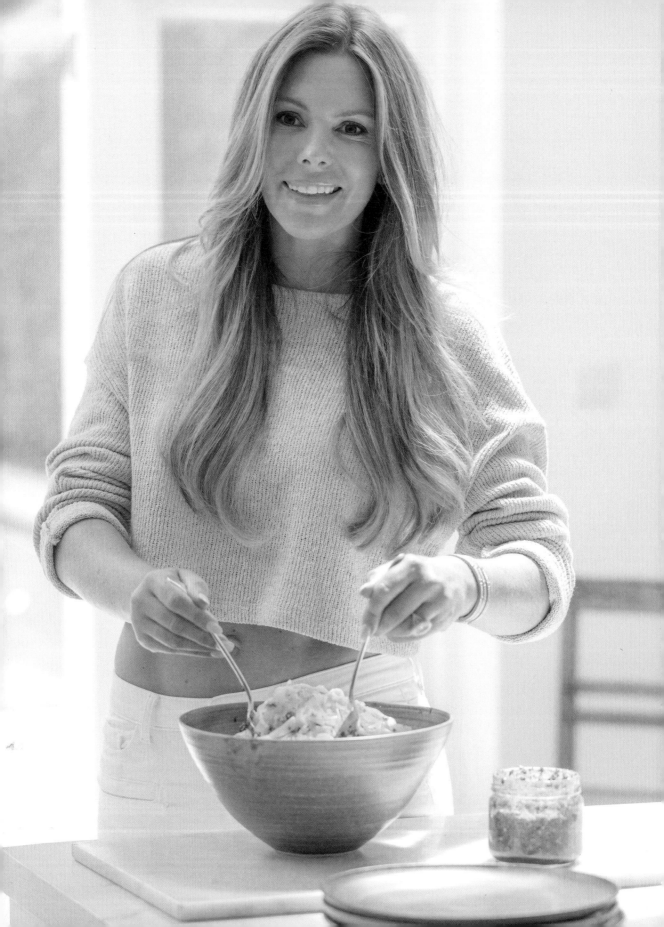

the *buddy* workout

get fit with family and friends for a healthier, happier you!

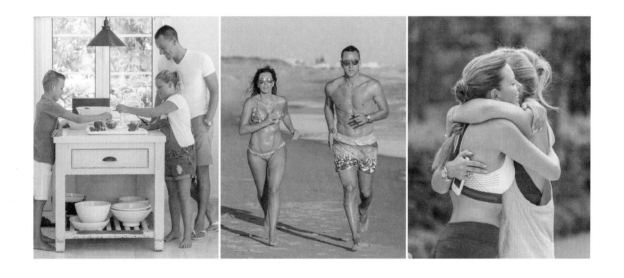

toni terry

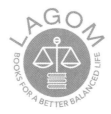

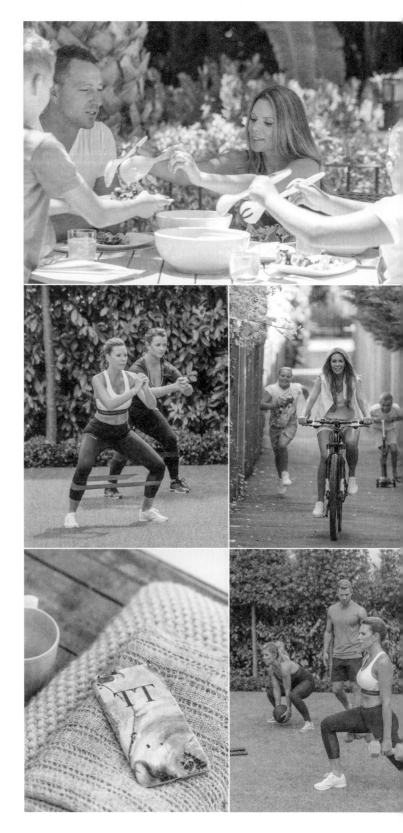

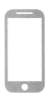

THE BUDDY WORKOUT APP

Go behind the scenes with Toni and unlock exclusive workouts and secret footage, from never-seen-before photos and recipe tutorials, to step-by-step exercises you can do alongside Toni!

To access all the exclusive content, download the free app from the iTunes App Store or Google Play Store, launch the app and point your device's camera at the pages with the special phone icon (above). All of Toni's tips and special features will then come to life on your screen!

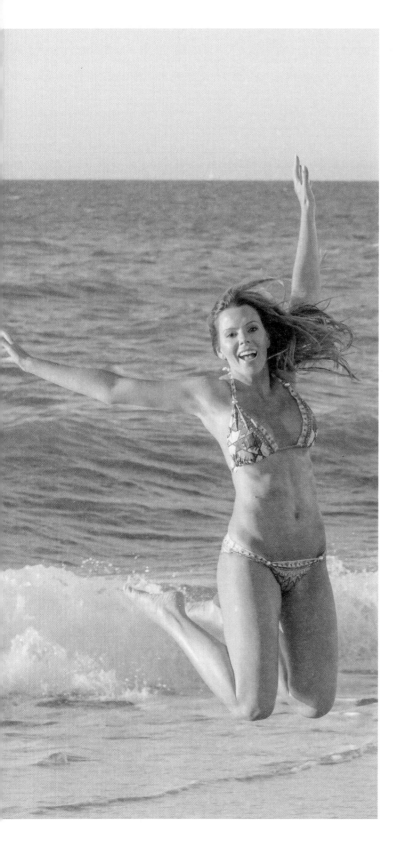

contents

“ I work out with Toni every week and I have to
say I really look forward to our sessions together.
We work really hard, motivate and push each other
through the hard stuff, but best of all we laugh – a lot.
Toni is the best workout buddy, totally inspirational
and a real friend. ”

Claire Fewings

“ Toni's been such a big motivation. She's helped me
on my weight loss journey by supporting me through our
training sessions with Bradley. We've now become workout
buddies and great friends. I love training together and
enjoying healthy, delicious food afterwards. ”

Connie Simmonds

66 Training with Toni has been an absolute pleasure. Right from the outset I could see that she was incredibly determined and up for a challenge. The key I believe for Toni is that she enjoys her workouts, varies the exercise she does, involves her family and friends, and, by eating healthily, keeps in fantastic shape. 99

Bradley Simmonds

66 We love being an active family and Toni has always been a great inspiration to me and our children Georgie and Summer. Toni has worked so hard to achieve her goals and I'm consistently in awe of how she's able to juggle family life with all of her training and other commitments. Being woken by the sound of the treadmill at 6am is a regular occurrence in the Terry household and she always makes sure we have a healthy breakfast before leaving for school or football. It's fantastic to see all of her hard work, enthusiasm and commitment to her health and fitness result in this book, one that I am sure will help inspire so many people. Toni is the perfect wife, mother and the rock of our family, and we are so proud of what she's achieved. 99

John Terry

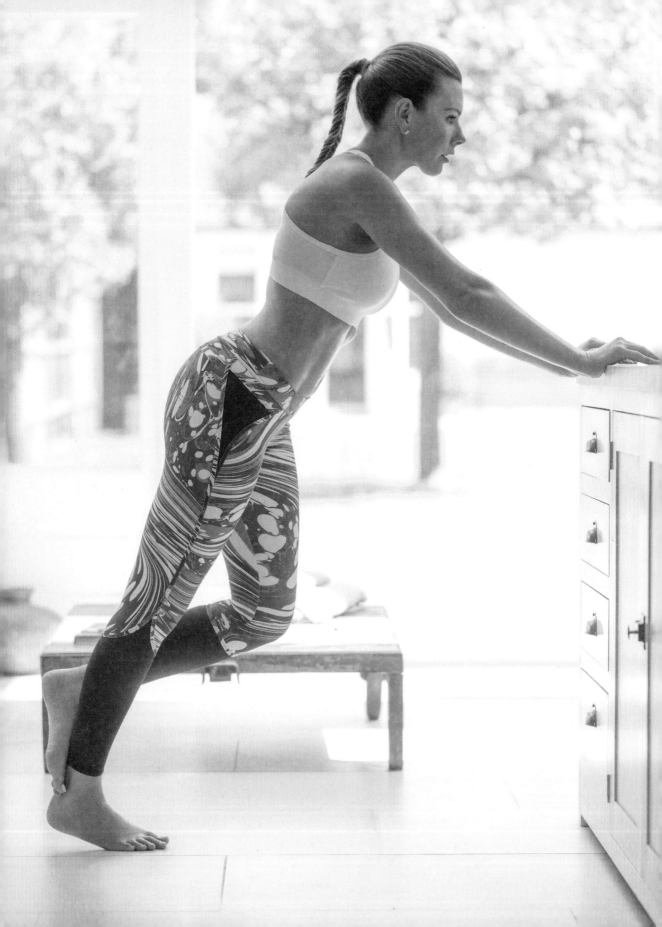

Keeping active and healthy has always been a big thing for me. It's been a constant throughout my life, keeping me focused and balanced. I've always been passionate about keeping fit and eating well – it makes me feel strong, confident and just happy, and who doesn't want that in their life!

introduction

As a child I was a bit of a tomboy and very sporty, and this proved my salvation when I was diagnosed with the back condition scoliosis as a teenager. Since then, I've tried to keep fit and I've always loved being outdoors. Now as a mum of two beautiful children, I'm constantly on the go and like nothing more than to get out and active with the family. Marriage to a high-profile footballer has, of course, taken me on an exciting journey in life, but living under the media spotlight does come with its own pressures. One of the main ones for me is the pressure to look good at all times – from public events where the cameras are flashing, to nipping out to the shops with newborn twins. It's always there.

Keeping fit and healthy not only helps me to look as good as I can, but I also feel stronger for it and it gives me confidence. However, it has taken me a long time to figure out what actually works. Like many people, I've tried all sorts of diets and exercise programmes, from punishing gym regimes to cutting down drastically on what I ate (which for me never worked). I am pretty determined when I put my mind to something, so I'm always totally committed to any new exercise or diet. But when I didn't see the results I wanted I'd find myself getting bored, or losing momentum, or just unable to stick to the impossible diets I'd devised for myself. And if you're pushing yourself to do something that frankly you'd prefer not to do, you really want a bit of payback at the end. Like a bit more definition to those arms, a boost in energy, a less squidgy bum perhaps – just *something* to show for all that hard work.

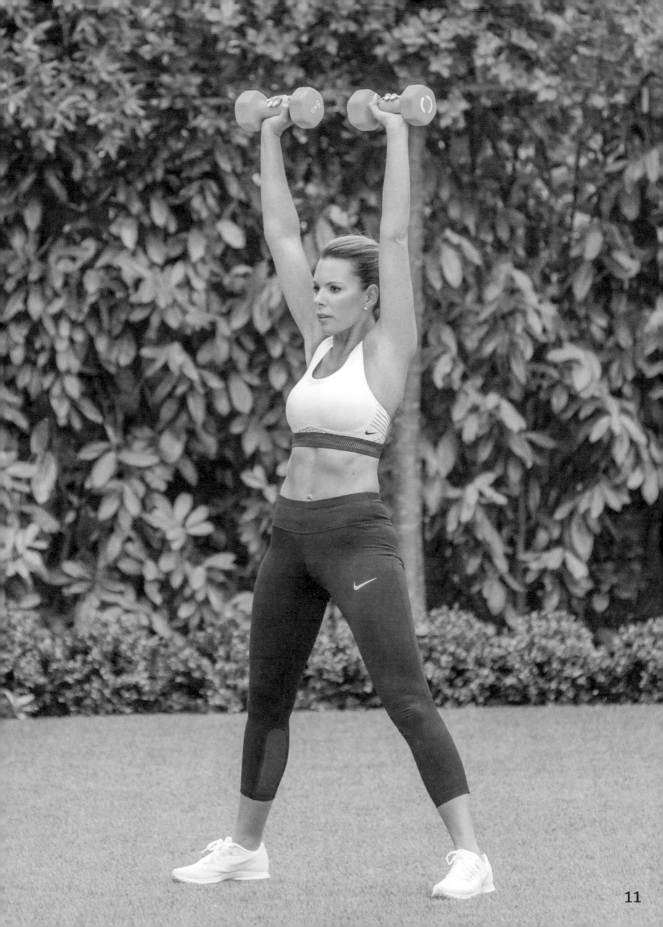

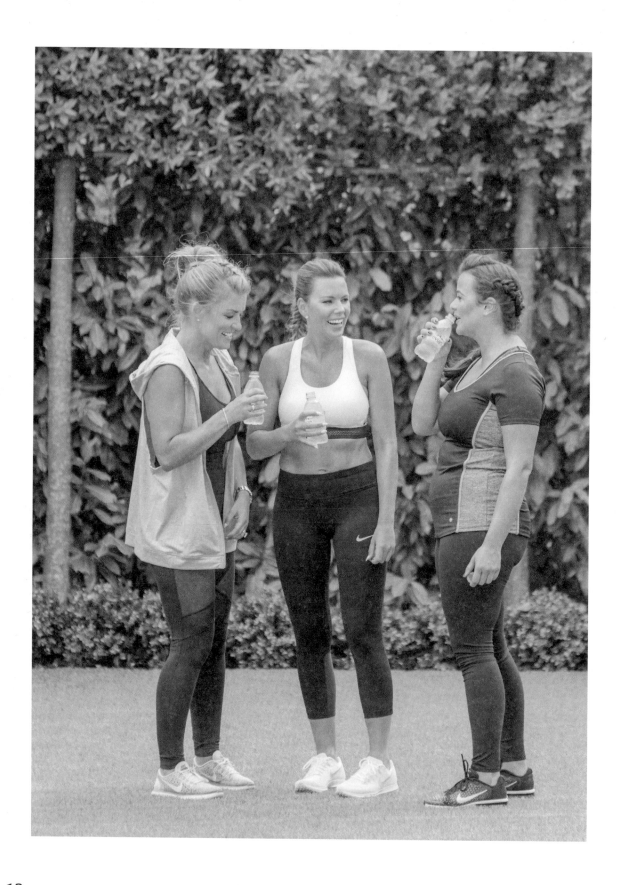

We then met regularly, pushed ourselves hard and had a huge amount of fun. Come rain or shine we were out there, always laughing, and motivating each other, all of us different sizes and shapes and fitness abilities.

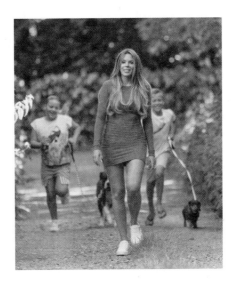

So what changed? What was the missing ingredient? And how did I start getting the results I always wanted? Well, it turned out to be something rather simple: people. John, still then captaining Chelsea, introduced me to a fitness trainer called Bradley Simmonds. Our first workout session involved the whole family, including my mum and dad. It was tough but really enjoyable and I remember we laughed from beginning to end. We were different fitness levels, ages crossing the generations, but we worked hard and had a great time.

This seemed to be a winning formula, so for my next training session with Bradley I invited a few friends over to work out with us. We then met regularly to exercise, pushed ourselves hard and had a huge amount of fun. The sessions seemed tough at the start but after two weeks became easier. Come rain or shine we were out there, always laughing, and motivating each other, all of us different sizes and shapes and fitness abilities. I'd finally hit upon a workout I loved – and I could see my body changing. Plus I also got to spend time with my buddies!

Since then I've always worked out with other people and developed a fitness programme that really produces results. I do a combination of cardio, HIIT and body weight training, and I have devised a set of exercises that can be done with partners, friends and on my own at home. On a daily basis, I also do the odd five-minute 'burst' workout from running up the stairs to squats in the kitchen – my family possibly think I'm a little mad but it helps to get results! In addition, I'm always out and about with my family cycling, walking, trampolining in the garden, or whatever takes our fancy.

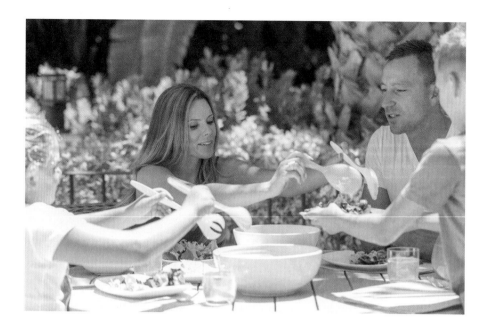

What you eat is also a key part in keeping fit and maintaining a healthy weight. Drastic dieting never worked for me – all that calorie counting and self-denial was unsustainable. Now I probably eat more than ever because I have balanced, nutritious meals, which I combine with exercise. I love to share breakfasts with my buddies after a tough workout as well as cook and eat good food with my family, and it's important to get the kids involved. What I love about exercise is that it gives you a healthy appetite; I enjoy food more and want my friends and family to love eating healthy food as much as I do. This book includes 35 of my favourite recipes, from gorgeous breakfasts and healthy snacks to filling evening meals that you can share with friends and family.

Alongside this, *The Buddy Workout* provides all the exercises that make up my weekly fitness programme, including specific partner workouts as well as exercises that can be done with a bunch of friends or alone. People of all fitness abilities can do these exercises at home with the minimum of equipment and fuss. There are step-by-step instructions, tips on how to keep motivated and how you too can train with others to get seriously fit and healthy. You don't need a fitness trainer to get you going, you just need this book, a bit of company and encouragement perhaps from friends and family, and a healthy dose of determination.

So grab some trainers, grab a buddy and get out there. No excuses!

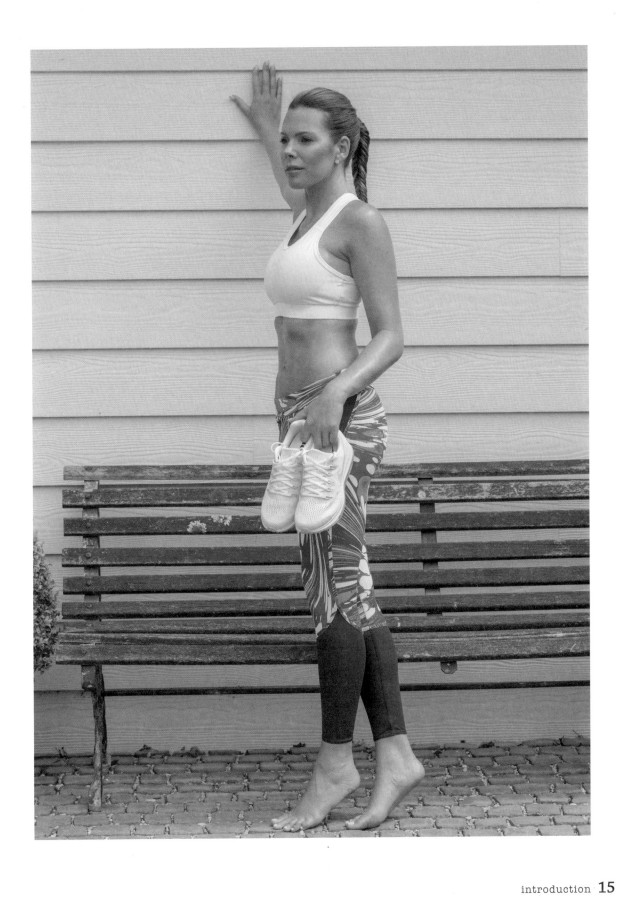

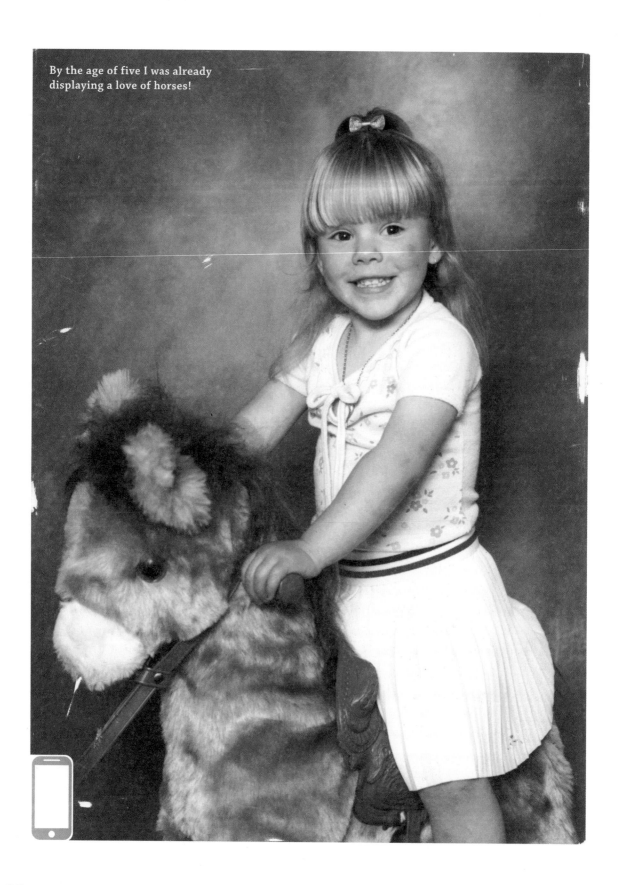

By the age of five I was already displaying a love of horses!

my journey

I've always been sporty and active, as far back as I can remember. As a child, I took up karate, earned my black belt at the age of eleven and ended up competing nationally, travelling all over the country with my parents who have constantly been incredibly supportive.

Then, at the age of 13, I went to a medical at school – it was just the normal check-up that everyone had. The nurse ran a few tests, and one of these was to touch my toes. As I did so, I remember her letting out a kind of a gasp, before saying she needed to speak to my parents. When I got home, my mum and dad asked to have a look at my back and it was then that we saw something we'd never noticed before. I had a huge lump on the right side of my back, from the shoulder right down to my waist. As they looked closer, they could also see that my left shoulder was lower than the right one, and on my chest, my left rib stuck out far more than the right side.

It was a huge shock for us, especially as it all seemed to have come out of the blue. We discovered eventually that I had scoliosis, a medical condition that causes an abnormal curve in the spine and usually develops in adolescence. I had a 75 per cent curve in my spine, shaped like a back-to-front S. The first consultant we saw told me to stop all exercise immediately, which, for a sporty 13-year-old, was devastating to hear. It was all so hard and I was suddenly really self-conscious about how I looked. Thankfully, my parents then took me to see another consultant and the treatment he suggested was the complete opposite: I should keep going with the exercise and be as flexible and agile as possible. I needed, however, to have an operation on my back otherwise the condition would get worse and I would likely end up in a wheelchair.

So we followed the advice of the second consultant and prepared for what turned out to be two operations. For a month prior to the first one I had to wear a back brace. To get fitted for it, I had a plaster cast made of my back and chest, and seeing it really upset me because I could see how misshapen I was.

The first eight-hour operation involved removing seven discs and one rib, which were placed in a freezer ready for the next operation seven days later. I was in intensive care for five days and in excruciating pain. In the next operation, the rib was shaved and used to replace the discs, and a titanium rod – which I still have to this day – was fused to my spine with wires. Then I was back in intensive care, followed by a two-week stay on a hospital ward to recover.

I had to lie flat and completely still for a total of four weeks. I've always been a bit of a fidget and by the end of that period I was desperate to get up and about! I begged the doctors to let me try and so they grudgingly allowed me to take a few steps. I have vivid memories of the day I managed to walk all around a pool table just in front of my bed – it took me about 20 minutes, mind! I'm told I made history that day as nobody had walked so quickly after the kind of operation I'd had. Seeing how determined I was, the hospital then allowed me to walk a bit every day.

When I eventually left hospital, my spine was much straighter and I had grown two inches but I had to continue to wear a huge back brace for six months. Going back to school was really tough – my self-confidence had plummeted. I could see other girls going out in skimpy tops to parties, whereas I just wanted to stay in and cover myself in a big jumper.

I was allowed to go back to karate. I kept active and my movement improved every day, and I found that the more I did, the more agile I became.

What helped to keep me sane, however, was that I was allowed to go back to karate, despite still needing to wear a back brace. I kept active and my movement improved every day, and I found that the more I did, the more agile I became. In fact, I progressed so well that I became British Kata Champion at 15, just a year after the operation. The doctors were really impressed – so much so that they wrote about my recovery to show that movement and exercise really could be the key to a faster recovery.

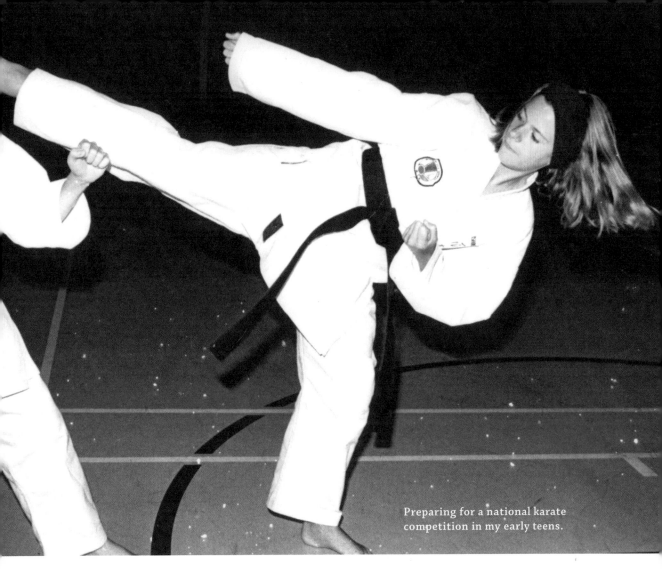

Preparing for a national karate competition in my early teens.

As a result I felt in control and more determined to keep as active as possible. Slowly, I got stronger, both physically and mentally, and now I can do pretty much whatever I want. I occasionally have to be a little careful with my back but there are only a couple of things I can't do: the crab and jumping out of a plane, two things I think a lot of adults have ruled out, back condition or not!

In truth, the scoliosis had more of long-term effect on my mental outlook, but in a positive way. Hard work and the support of my family and friends got me through it, and now, if ever I'm tired or unhappy about something, I tell myself to stop whinging and just get on with it. It toughened me a little and made me more determined – traits that have proved useful over the years. After that first medical scare, life settled back into normality. By my late teens

> To begin with, it was all quite scary – wherever we went John would be recognised, and the press were everywhere.

I was doing the kind of normal stuff teens do and I had a good bunch of friends. When I was 18 I went along to a nightclub with a few pals and it was there that I met John. At the time he was playing for Chelsea's youth team, but I don't think he even mentioned he was a footballer that night. To be honest, I didn't have the first clue about football – I didn't come from a family who followed it, and when he first told me what he did I didn't really think anything of it.

In any case, we took a shine to each other and ended up dating. I had a good job in London at the time and, as a youth player, John was on around £38 a week, so I was the main breadwinner in those days. John used to run me to the train station when I was commuting and even had dinner on the table for me at the end of day – he's a very good cook! He'd sometimes leave little cards for me on my car window or give me flowers – all very romantic.

Within a few months of us meeting, John made his full debut as a player at Chelsea and started to become better known. It still hadn't really hit home with me until I was at karate training one night, and suddenly saw him on television. I couldn't believe it! As John's football career progressed, both at Chelsea and as an England player from 2003, public interest in him just grew and grew. To begin with, it was all quite scary – wherever we went he'd be recognised, and the press were everywhere. We were photographed more and more, and amid the glitterati of the sporting world, I (former karate champ and tomboy from Essex) felt like a bit of an alien.

In 2002, we decided to try for a baby. This proved more difficult than we'd anticipated as I had developed polycystic ovaries, which can affect fertility. After a long three years, just one cycle of an IUI fertility treatment resulted in us conceiving a child, and we were thrilled. Six weeks into the pregnancy, we discovered I was carrying twins – John was overjoyed and I was too, if a little daunted by the prospect of two babies!

A week before the babies were due, John had to go to an England training camp in Portugal in preparation for the FIFA World Cup 2006. I had insisted

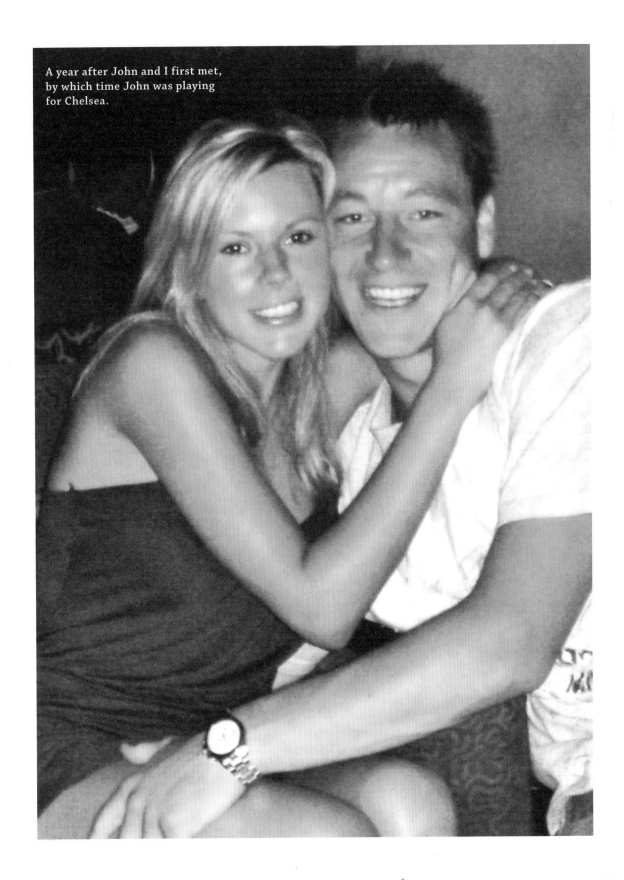

A year after John and I first met, by which time John was playing for Chelsea.

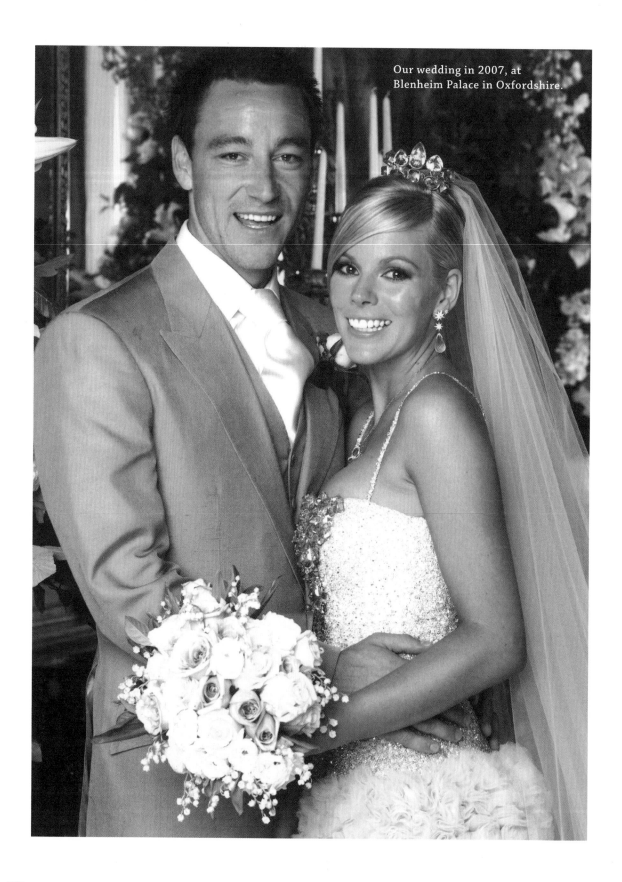

Our wedding in 2007, at Blenheim Palace in Oxfordshire.

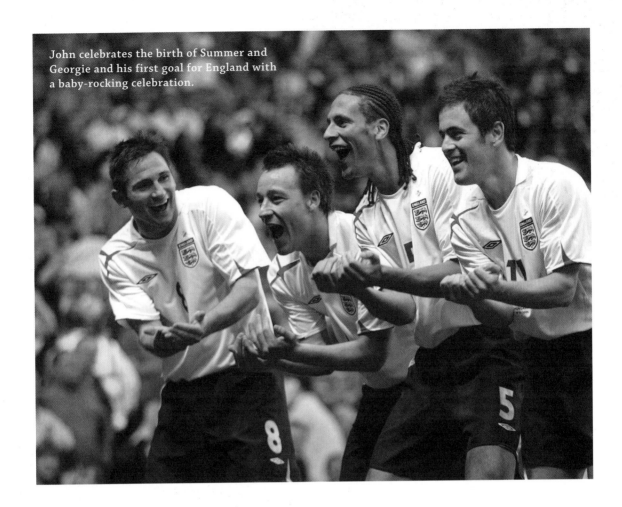

John celebrates the birth of Summer and Georgie and his first goal for England with a baby-rocking celebration.

he go as the scans were all fine and the C-section wasn't booked until the following week. The night after he went, however, the babies (as they so often do) had other plans and I started to go into labour. John of course made immediate preparations to fly back. My contractions came on fast and by the time I arrived at the hospital in London, they were every four minutes. Despite this, I was still determined that the babies weren't going to come as John hadn't got there yet! Nonetheless, I was rushed into theatre and the babies, my beloved Georgie and Summer, were delivered. As soon as I could I phoned John who had just landed. He was really emotional, crying down the phone, and a passenger at the airport gave John a handkerchief, something I still have to this day.

Less than a month after the babies had arrived, John was back playing for England, this time in Germany for the FIFA World Cup. I joined him there

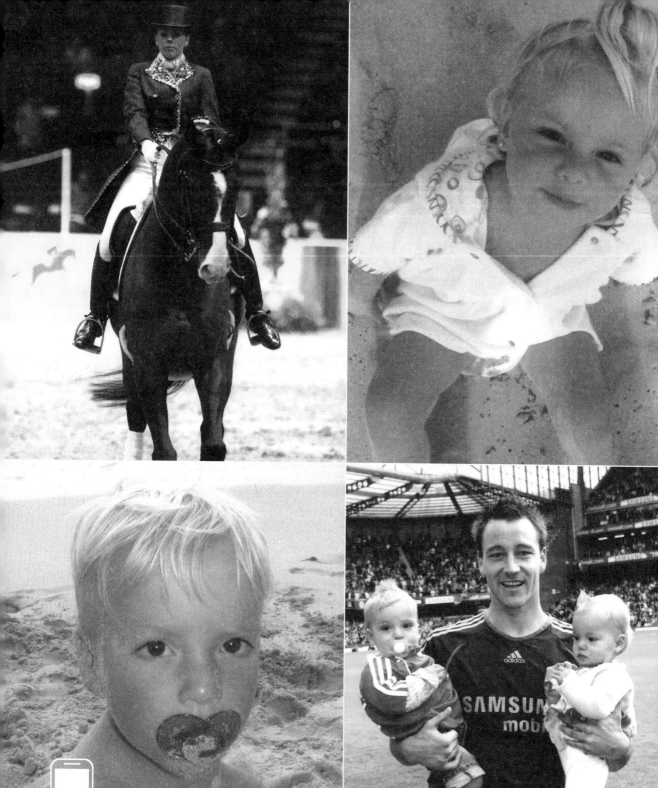
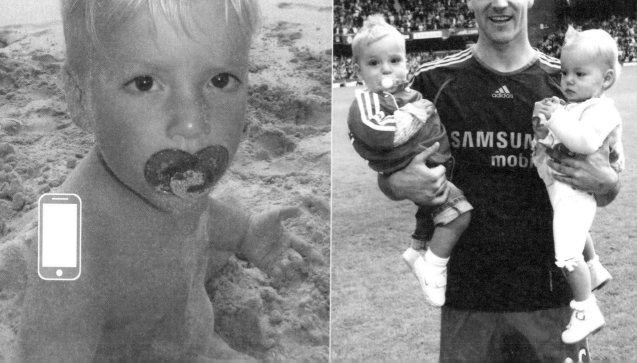

with the newborns and the media interest in us and all the players was huge – we were photographed constantly. Everyone else seemed to look amazing, but I just hated all the pictures I saw of me. Perhaps I should have been easier on myself – I had just had twins after all! – but this was the slightly insane world I lived in and the pressure was immense. In the main I wanted to feel good about myself again, and I knew I had the ability to do something about it. As a result, I went on a six-week detox diet and managed to lose two stone. I actually ate loads during this time but it was all very green, lean food and I felt great. It gave me the kick-start I needed and I could see how eating well could make you feel really energised – and I needed all the energy I could get with twins! This spurred me on to get fitter and I went along to a gym. I took the usual induction, and sessions involved running on the treadmill for about half an hour and doing a few machines. I did that for a couple of years but I didn't feel it was me and I found it all pretty boring.

I actually ate loads during this time but it was all very green, lean food and I felt great. It gave me the kick-start I needed and I could see how eating well could make you feel really energised.

At the same time, I started exercising at home with the babies. I'd do squats, sit-ups and stretches on the floor next to them, and all sorts of stuff, and we'd always end up giggling. I think they loved watching me jump around, looking a little ridiculous! Lifting the babies, I noticed quite a difference in my arms, which spurred me on to do more of these mini-workouts. My mum would join in and we'd gently lift the babies in circles, as well as go swimming, walking and I'd also run with the buggy.

When the kids were at nursery I took up dressage with horses, which to this day I love. It looks like you're just sitting there on a horse, but it actually gives you a real workout. It's great for your core as you have to hold yourself in a certain way on horseback, and a strong core puts less pressure on the back. I was also ploughing on with my twice-weekly gym workouts but not really getting anywhere with them, so I decided to change tack and work out with a personal trainer. We worked out together, just the two of us, but again I found it dull after a while – something was missing and I wasn't sure what it was.

I was then introduced to HIIT (which stands for high-intensity interval training) by the trainer Joe Wicks. This involves quick bursts of intense exercise followed by short periods of recovery. I did that for a year, four days a week, and I got totally addicted. This was far more my style of workout: I loved the intensity of it and I could easily fit a quick 20-minute session into my day. I had a lot going on with the twins and the horses, as well as the demands of John's career, but it got to the point that it didn't matter what I was doing that day, I would get up a little earlier or just find that 20 minutes. I'd sometimes work out with John if he was around, but again I was often exercising on my own and, although I felt I'd found a workout that suited me, I was still not quite as fully engaged with it as I would have liked.

We all had busy lives, filled with family and work, but this was friends time, a regular morning get-together when we'd turn the music up and get exercising.

The light-bulb moment came when John invited a trainer called Bradley round to the house one Sunday morning. The plan was that I'd be training with him on my own, but as John, my mum and dad and the kids were all at home, we thought we'd try working out together. When John said to Bradley, 'Listen, mate, I know you're meant to be here for Toni but would you mind training the whole family?', Bradley took it very well! The resulting workout session was so much fun. It was hard, and we obviously had to vary the exercises depending on our different abilities, but we didn't stop laughing!

So Bradley was obviously a winner and I was keen to invite him back and continue with those workout sessions. The thought of training with him on my own was a bit daunting, however, particularly as I'd never trained with a man before. So, for a bit of Dutch courage, I texted and called some of my girlfriends, telling them about Bradley and inviting them over for a training session. Five of them came and we tried some circuit training in the garden. The girls were at different levels of fitness and had their own reasons and goals for wanting to train. And they were all very different personalities – I'm quite motivated and strict with myself whereas some of my friends need more encouragement, shall we say!

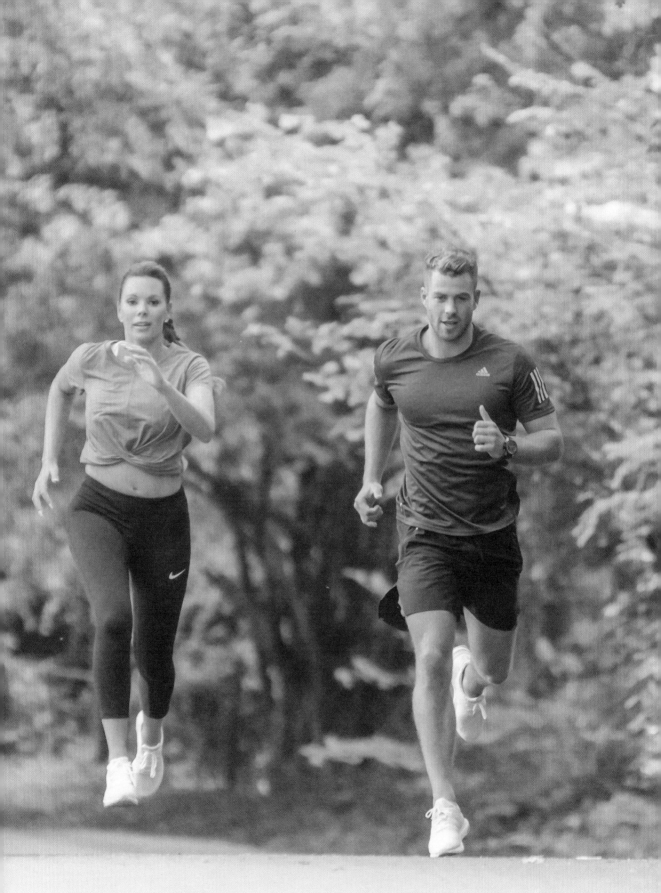

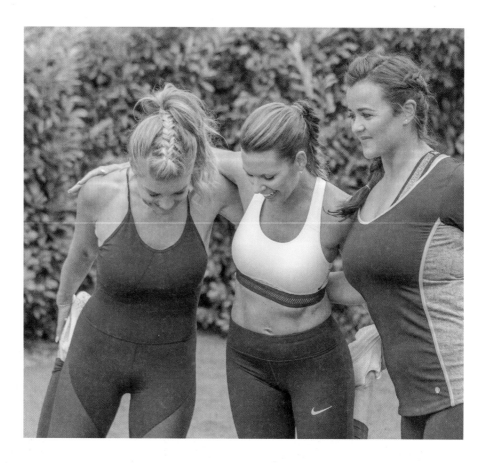

Despite all these differences, however, we all loved the session and continued working out together. We all had busy lives, filled with family and work, but this was friends time, a regular morning get-together when we'd turn the music up and get exercising, whether it was pouring with rain or bright sunshine. For variety, we'd work out in each other's gardens and whoever's turn it was would do breakfast – perhaps a protein shake or pancake. It was a social thing, we'd exercise for an hour, then spend half an hour catching up. The time just flew by and we'd almost forget that we were exercising – a total win/win situation.

These days I always get together with my friends to work out around twice a week. I also work out with a trainer or with John if he's around, I exercise on my own, and I do all sorts of activities with the family. I love the variety and, when I'm training at home, my friends know that my house and garden is always open. It's a system that I can fit into a busy day, it really produces results and I feel happier and more confident. You've got to try it!

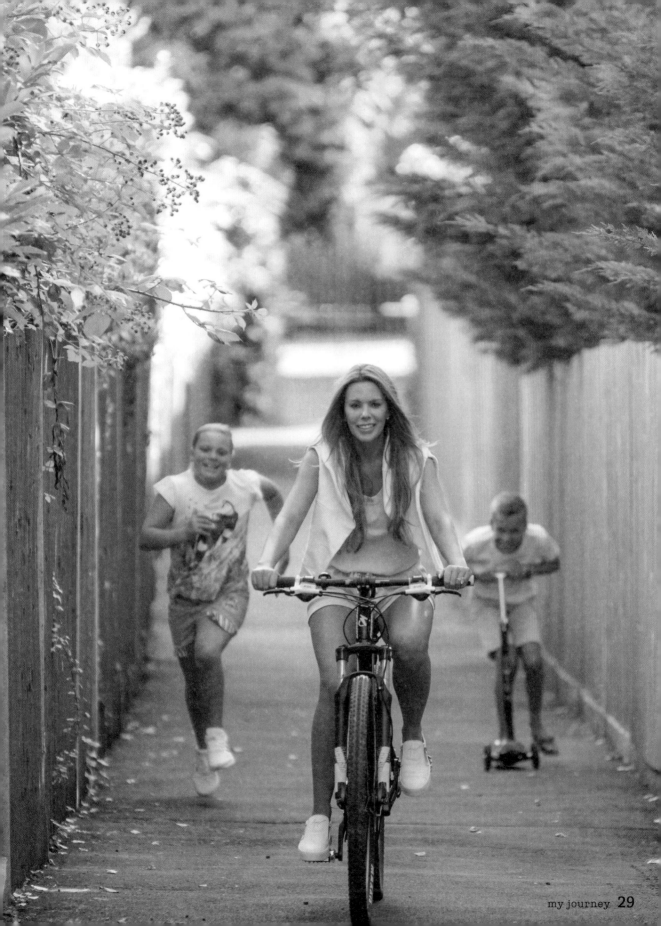

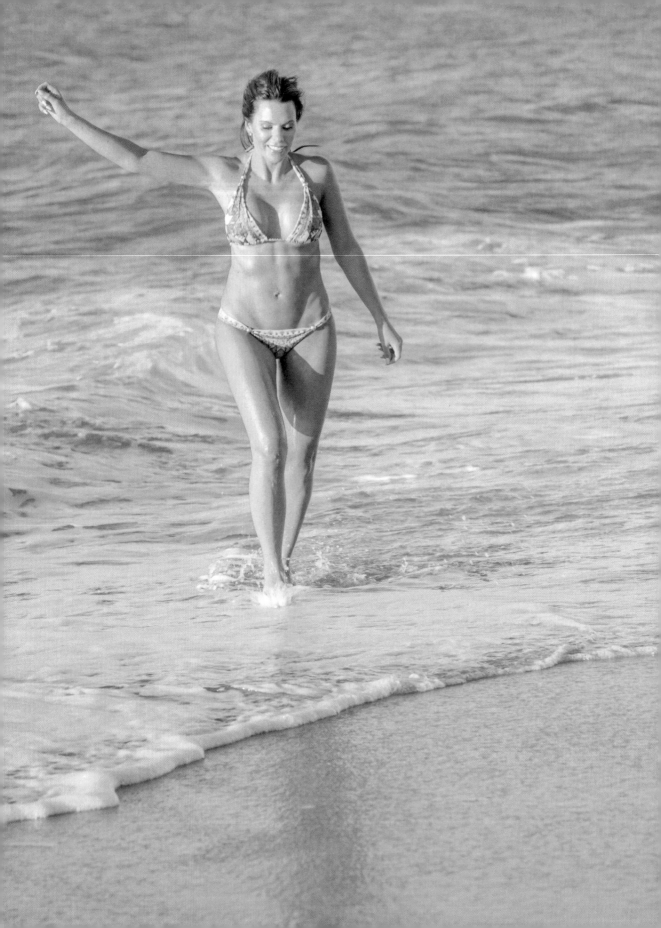

Getting fit and healthy is about doing what you enjoy and figuring out what works for you. You need also to focus on what you want to achieve, keep motivated and encourage those around you. Eating well and exercising with your buddies not only does wonders for your body but also makes for a happy life.

live

setting goals

When you embark on any new fitness regime or healthy lifestyle, it's a good idea to set goals because they help you to keep going and add a bit of structure to your workout programme. Over the years, my reasons for exercising have changed, but I've always worked towards goals, however small. I love the challenge and it's a great feeling when you achieve them and get the results you've always wanted. Here are my top tips for setting goals in your fitness and health journey.

● Keep your goals specific and start with small ones at first and build from there. It might be that you aim to drink more water, do a certain set of squats or eat healthier breakfasts, but keep in mind that smaller goals are easier to achieve and will keep you motivated for longer.

● Have a variety of aims that you can work towards in the short- and long-term. You might want to achieve something specific like plank jacks by the end of the week, or gain a bit of muscle definition after three months, but it's good to have a mixture of aims to keep you motivated.

● Be realistic and don't set yourself such ambitious goals that you'll never be able to achieve them. There's only so much you can do with your body shape: you won't instantly lose stones of weight or get taller. Changing your body outline takes time and a lot of commitment.

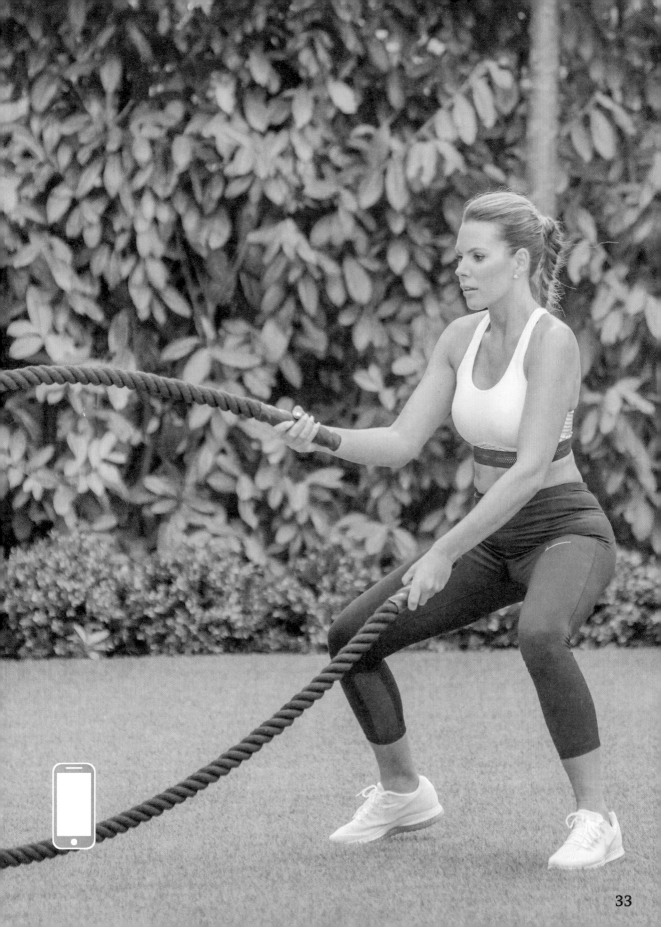

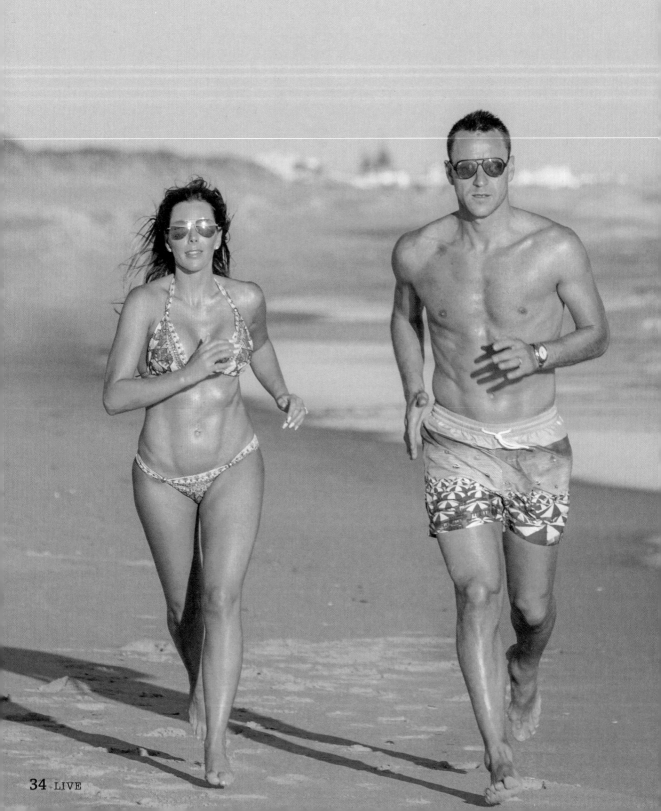

Keep positive and set goals that also focus on how your feel, rather than on bits of your body that you hate.

● Think about what you can realistically do in a day or week. How busy are you and what else do you need to fit in your day? I'll look at my week ahead and try to think in advance when I can exercise or whether I need to prepare some healthy food for when I'm out and about.

● Stick to your commitments to work out with your buddies and schedule it in to your day or week. Arrange a specific time to meet up and get going on time if you can – there's always time for chat afterwards! I often find that the morning is the best time to exercise, especially when I have a busy day ahead as I know it's done and it sets me up for the day nicely.

● Tell your friends and family what your goals are. (As soon as I tell anyone what I'm aiming for, such as I'm going to run 10k in 45 minutes, that's it, I've got to do it!) For some people, it works if they actually write down their goals and put them somewhere public where they'll see them every day, like on the fridge door or a computer monitor.

● Keep positive and set goals that also focus on how you feel, rather than on bits of your body that you hate. Succeeding in any exercise programme is all about having the right mindset and if you feel good about what you're doing then you're more likely to keep going. Don't just focus on what you CAN'T do or eat, but what you CAN do and eat – like running up those stairs without getting out of breath or discovering a new food or recipe that you love. Write down your achievements, however small, so you see how far you've progressed and congratulate yourself and those around you.

keeping motivated

Working out with a partner or your buddies is obviously one of the best ways to keep motivated. But there are a host of other things you can do to achieve the goals you've set yourself and to keep committed in the long term. Here are a few things that have helped me to keep going.

● If you're a beginner or just starting out on your journey, start slowly with fewer training sessions and see how you go. Keep your workouts short – don't straightaway blitz it for two hours and then suffer the next day. You can build on the regularity and length of your sessions once your body has got used to a new way of working.

● Encourage your friends or workout partner and they'll do the same for you. Remind them of their goals, how they felt at the start of the journey and how fantastic they'll feel if they smash through their goals.

● Track your progress. Work to a timeframe – for example, 'I want to workout X many times over the next two weeks, and in three months I want to achieve X.' Create a schedule and record how long each session was and how you coped, and look back over your comments. A month down the line you might be surprised at the progress you've made.

Encourage your friends or workout partner and they'll do the same for you. Remind them of their goals, how they felt at the start of the journey.

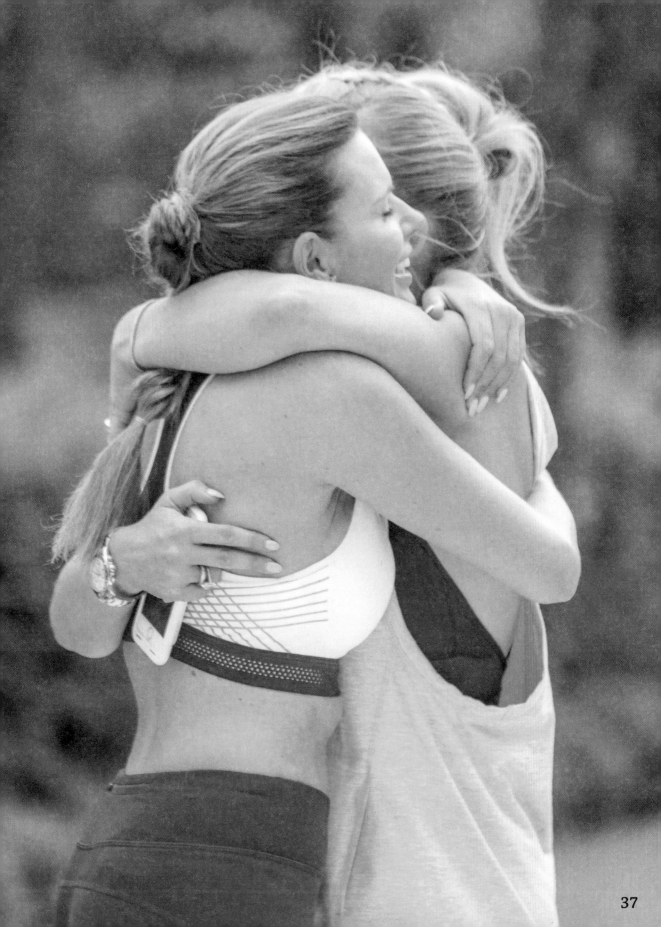

Rest and recover between sessions. You need to get the most out of each workout and if you want to keep going over the long term you need to avoid injury and burnout.

● As you track your progress, think about how you feel and notice any changes in your body or skin. I don't weigh myself but I will sometimes take photos of myself in a bikini or similar clothing over a set period of time to see if there's any difference in my body outline and definition. Often my clothes will just feel different and I'll know that my shape's changing. Look also at your skin, hair and nails as these are often a good indicator of your general health. When I exercise my skin positively glows and I feel the benefit of it for hours afterwards.

● Rest and recover between sessions. You need to get the most out of each workout and if you want to keep going over the long term you need to avoid injury and burnout. Your body may well ache a bit a day or two after a workout but total exhaustion or pain will stop you in your tracks. You want to feel great and energised so that you'll keep going towards your goals.

● Recognise that there will be days when you lack a little energy or just don't feel up to it. Often you can push through it and working out will make you feel a lot better. The benefit of workout buddies is that they can instantly lift your mood, share their worries and experiences, and get you through the difficult days. If you have to miss a day, don't fret about it. Life can be unpredictable, just pick things up again the next day and keep motivated.

● Pump up the music. Working out to music can really help to put you in just the right mood for exercise. When I exercise with my friends, we'll take turns in providing the music, which is always a bit of a talking point and adds to the fun of our sessions together.

● If you lose a bit of momentum or enthusiasm for your workout, try something new. This doesn't mean you have to start a whole new activity, you might just need to tweak your routine, add a new exercise or set yourself a new challenge. Small changes can make all the difference and your buddies might have some ideas about what's worked for them.

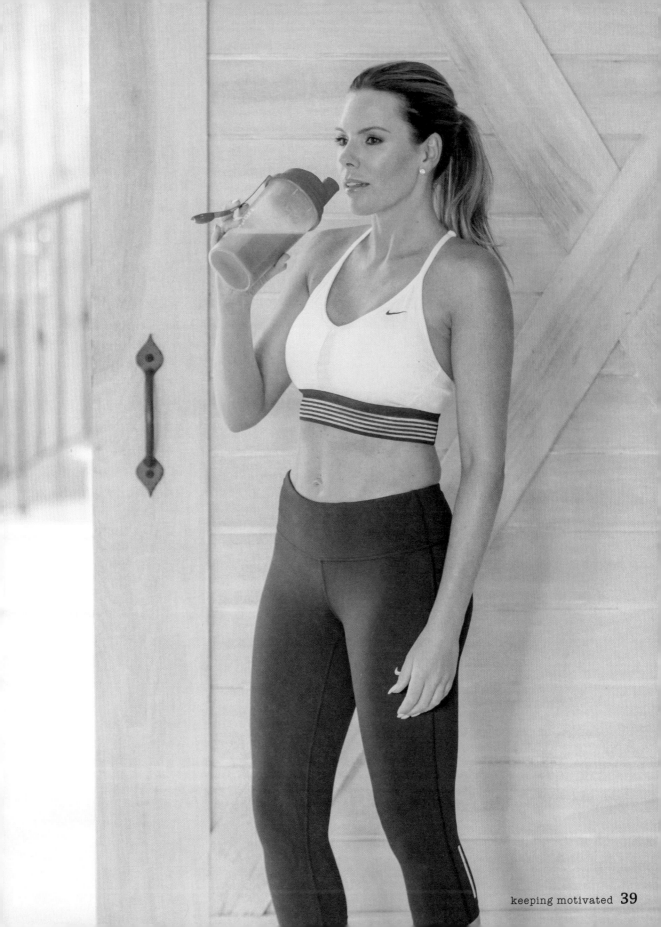

why buddy up?

As we've already seen, there are so many benefits to working out with a buddy, whether you're doing specific partner-workout exercises (see page 76) or you're just getting together with others to do your weekly workout. Here are just a few more reasons why exercising with a buddy makes sense.

1 FUN!
Working out with others is just more fun, especially when you're with people whose company you enjoy. It gives you an excuse to catch up with friends on a regular basis, have a bit of a laugh and bond as you grit your teeth and get through one more push up! It's also a great way to spend time with a partner or a family member away from the usual distractions of work, school and screens, and the madness of everyday life. Kids usually love to get out and play games – they have a natural sense of fun that us adults need to tap into a bit more! And if you're having fun working out with a bunch of people you like, time really does fly past and before you know it your workout will be done and you can get on with your day.

2 COMMITMENT
If you're on your own it's so much easier to bail if you've had a bad day or are just not feeling up to it. It's much harder to ditch your workout if you've made a commitment to exercise with others. If you don't want to let your workout buddies down you'll find that extra reserve of energy you didn't know you had, and chances are you'll feel more energetic afterwards, not to mention virtuous.

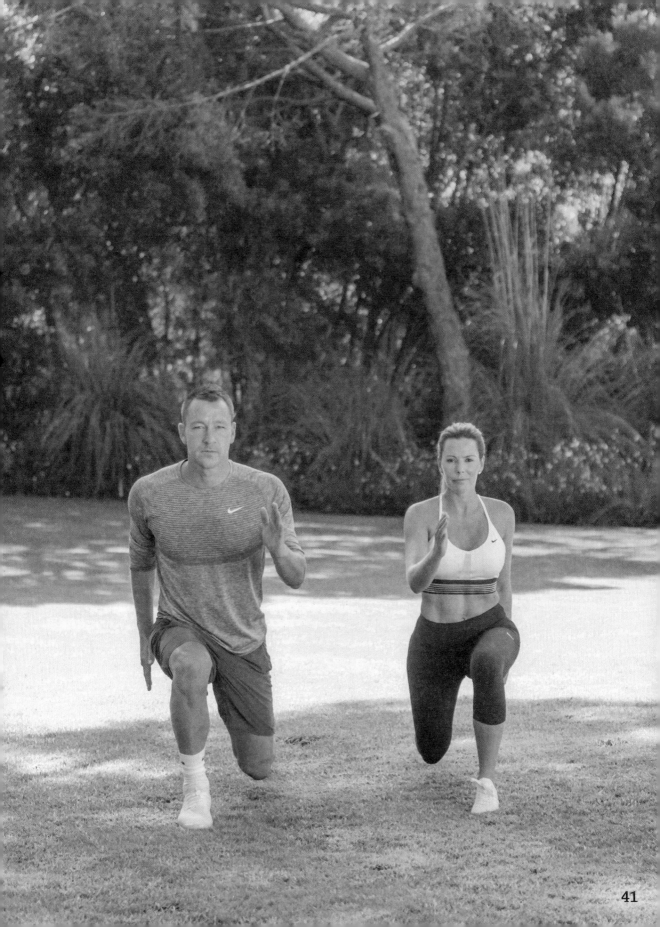

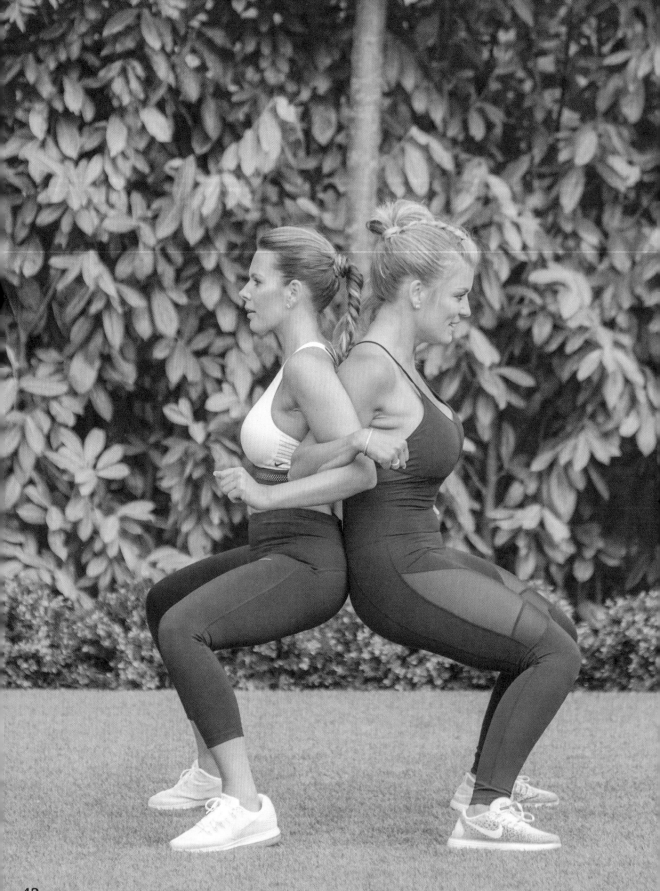

3 CONFIDENCE

Starting out on any fitness or lifestyle programme can be daunting, but if you have a buddy or two supporting you, the process can be far less intimidating. Once you've started on your fitness journey, the right buddy will help you to give it your all and really get the results you want. It's like having your own personal cheerleader! Evidence shows that working out with a buddy increases the effectiveness of your exercise and you're far less likely to give up weeks down the line. The right workout buddy will help you to reach your goals and push you to do those few extra reps. Exercising is all about having the right mindset and if you've got a pal celebrating your achievements, however small, then it'll keep you positive and boost your confidence.

I tried to encourage one of my friends to make the most of her workouts in the build up to her wedding. On the day she looked amazing, and she said my encouragement really motivated her. She does exactly the same for me on days when I'm tired or just not a hundred per cent. I know for sure that my friends and family help me to reach my goals: if I've told them that I'm going to do something, that's it, I've got to do it, no question!

4 VARIETY

On your own, it's easy to get stuck in a rut and do the same routine day in day out, which never bodes well for sticking to your workout in the long term. With buddies, you're much more likely to do something new. They might have some ideas about new elements you can introduce into your workout or inspire you to try something different. Your buddies are likely to have different skills and knowledge from which you can benefit. For me, the key to sticking to any exercise is to keep it varied, to try new things and to keep working towards different goals.

5 COMPETITION

A little healthy rivalry between friends and family is no bad thing. If your workout buddy is a little fitter than you, it might motivate you to work harder, especially if they're giving you lots of encouragement. And when you're with others of all abilities you're much more likely to exercise properly, doing those squats as they should be done, rather than just going through the motions.

Exercising is all about having the right mindset and if you've got a pal celebrating your achievements, however small, then it'll keep you positive.

Remember, a good workout partner should make exercise fun, not the opposite! It really helps if they are encouraging, with a positive attitude.

6 SAFETY

If you're out in public, many people feel safer if they're with someone, especially if they're running at night or in an isolated environment. In any workout, a buddy will also be there to spot if you're doing a move wrong or to help with balance.

THE RIGHT BUDDY

What makes for the best kind of workout buddy? Someone you like, who you don't want to let down, and whose company you enjoy. Remember, a good workout partner should make exercise fun, not the opposite! It really helps if they are encouraging, with a positive attitude – the last thing you want is someone whinging throughout the whole session, dragging you and everyone else down with them. Your workout buddies can be a different size, shape or gender, and they might be exercising for all sorts of different reasons, but it helps if you're not totally mismatched. A beginner just starting out on their fitness journey might feel a little intimidated by someone training for the Olympics. Saying that, for some people that might be just the inspiration they need, so whatever floats your boat!

SOCIAL MEDIA

Some people might find it a little tricky to find that perfect workout buddy or group of like-minded pals. If so, that's not a problem as many people use social media to find someone to exercise with – there are lots of sites out there that can help (see page 256). You can also chat with online communities if you don't want to bore your friends with that new exercise or recipe you've just tried. You can compare the highs and lows of exercise and celebrate achievements – it's amazing how a positive comment from someone you hardly know can really boost your confidence. You can also discover new exercises and pass on what you've learnt to others. My instagram page (@toniterry26) shows me exercising, shares other people's buddy success stories and I hope provides some inspiration for those starting out.

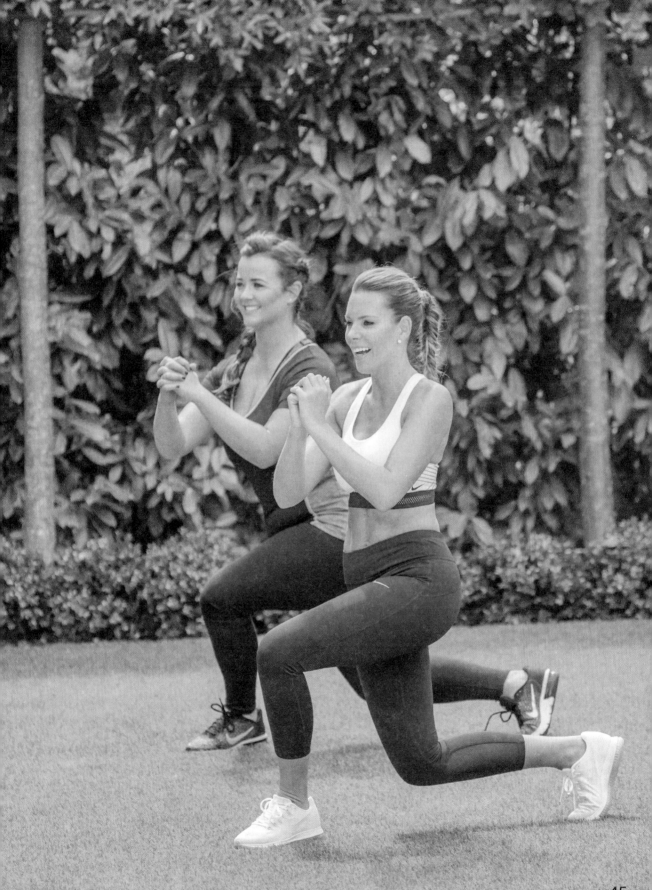

get that glow

When it comes to my appearance and skincare routine, I tend to keep things fairly simple. For the everyday, I'm all about a fresh, natural look, but I will then go for something more glam if I'm out at a special event. I'm a firm believer that if you're fit and healthy and eating nutritious foods, it will show in your appearance – you'll simply radiate beauty and strength. Saying that, sometimes we could all do with a little help to achieve that 'healthy glow' so here are a few simple tricks I've learnt over the years.

WATER

I try to drink at least two litres of water every day and more if I'm somewhere hot or working out hard. It really is important to keep hydrated if you want to keep your energy levels up, maintain a healthy weight and keep your skin radiant looking and fresh. First thing in the morning and at night, I also like to have a cup of hot water with a slice of fresh lemon. It's a wonderful cleanser for the body, helping to flush out toxins, reduce acidity and aid digestion, and it's much healthier than lots of coffee and tea which can be so dehydrating. I'm also a big fan of coconut water – despite being sweet, it's low in sugars and contains lots of calcium and minerals. It's great for rehydrating the body and for regulating the body temperature after a workout.

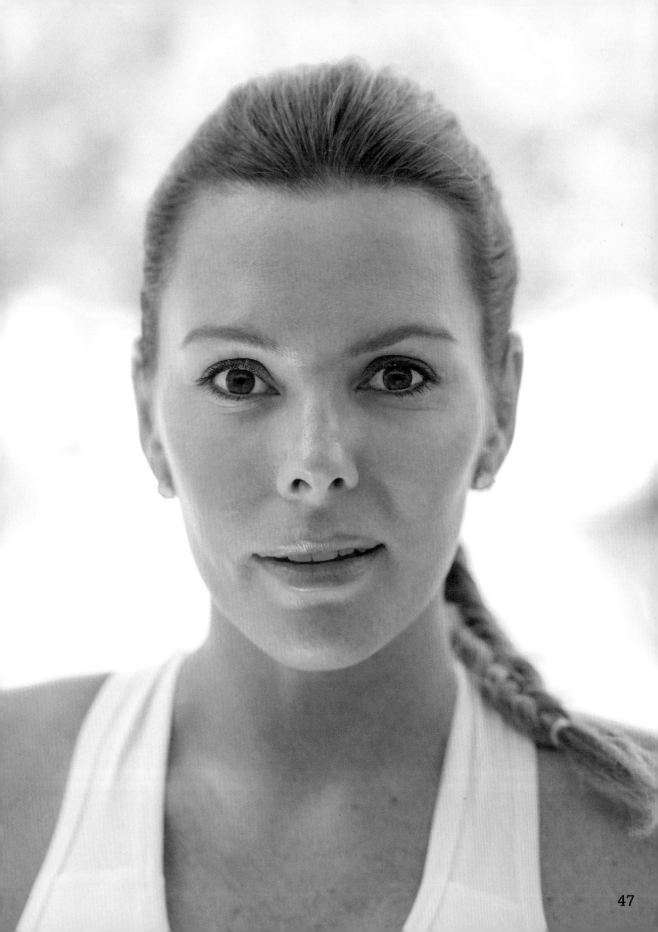

If you eat lots of fruit and vegetables, get outside every day, eat a healthy and varied diet and drink plenty of water, you should get the vast majority of nutrients you need for a healthy body and radiant skin.

SKIN

I wear factor 50 sun protection on my face every day. I'm outdoors a lot and fortunate enough to live in Portugal part of the year so I'm careful with the sun. Too much exposure to the rays is of course dangerous and incredibly ageing for the skin. If you want tanned skin, it's so much healthier to apply a bit of bronzer to the face or body. For my cheeks and face I'll often use a bronzing stick – there are so many good ones out there which will even out and hydrate the surface of the skin and give you that summer glow.

Throughout the year, I use a foaming facial scrub morning and night, which cleanses and gently exfoliates the skin. I also use products containing retinol, which unclogs pores, smooths the skin and evens out skin discoloration. (A very small percentage of people with sensitive skin can't use retinol cream or retinoids, so do be careful and test a little bit before you use it.) Every now and then I have a glycolic acid peel, a type of exfoliant that is really good for evening my complexion and a little bit of pigmentation I have on my skin. Again, anyone with really sensitive skin should be careful here. I also use a body scrub about twice a week, a good hydrating moisturiser and some body oil containing vitamin E.

I don't take any supplements as I try to get all the nutrients and vitamins I need from the food and drink I have. Saying that, during the winter months when most people are exposed to less sunlight, vitamin D supplements are a good idea. Otherwise, I'm a firm believer that if you eat lots of fruit and vegetables, get outside every day, eat a healthy and varied diet and drink plenty of water, you should get the vast majority of nutrients you need for a healthy body and radiant skin. A really good workout gets the blood pumping, and I find my skin glows for hours afterwards.

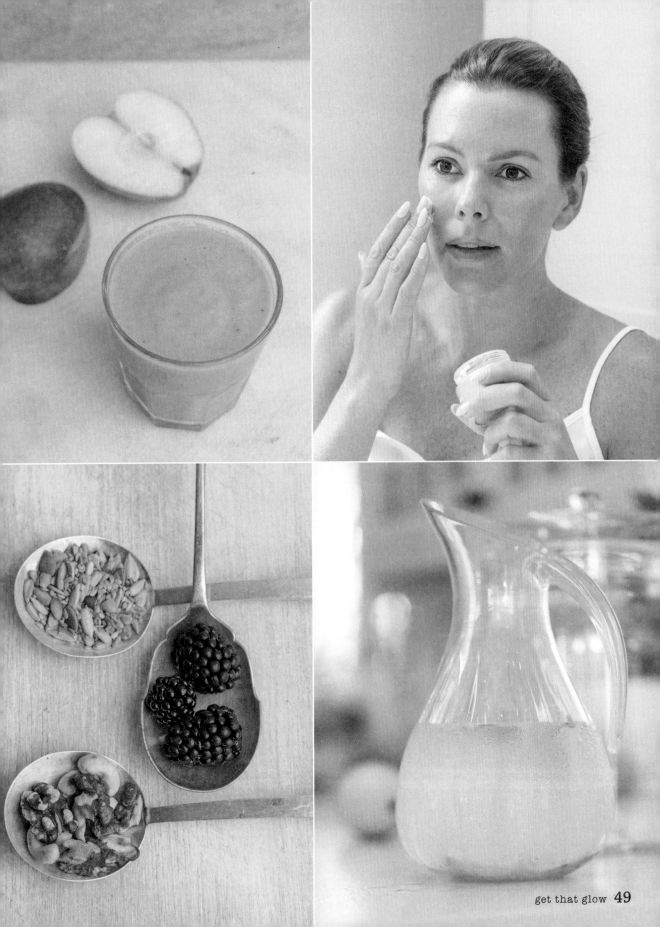

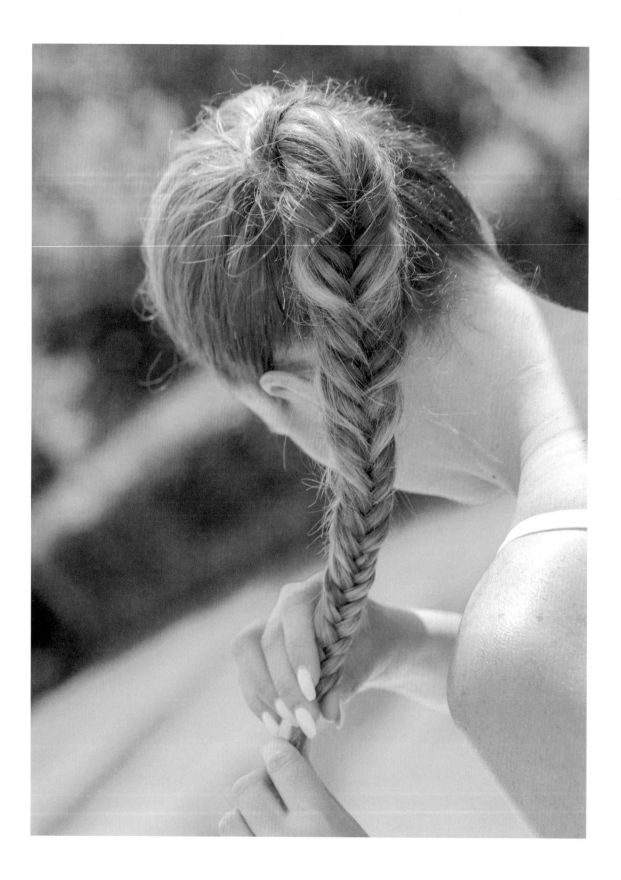

HAIR

Again, a nutritious diet full of healthy proteins, omega fatty acids (found in oily fish and plant sources like avocado and walnuts) along with lots of vegetables, berries and fruit will help to improve the health of your hair. Saying that, our hair often has to put up with a lot – sun, exercise and the products we put on it all take their toll – so there's plenty you can do to improve its condition and overall look.

Regular cuts are a must and I wash it every other day, as washing every day can strip your hair of its natural oils, dry the scalp and result in less healthy looking hair. Every couple of weeks I'll use a hair scrub, which helps to remove any build-up of products and is good for the scalp. In hot weather, I'll also wear a product to protect my hair from the sun and heat and occasionally I'll put conditioner on my hair, plait it and sleep with it on overnight. This gives my hair a deep-condition and it always feels softer and more moisturised the next day.

PHOTOS

Photos and selfies are now so much part of everyday life that we could all do with tips on how to look our best on camera. I've learnt that I definitely have a good side, and I'll often look longer and leaner if I stand side-on when someone's taking a photo, as standing square-on can sometimes be a little unflattering. I've also recently learnt that a little bit of oil on your limbs looks really good on camera. My top tip, however, is just to relax and smile – tense and moody does not make a good picture and people just look more naturally radiant when they're happy!

Our hair often has to put up with a lot – sun, exercise and the products we put on it – so there's plenty you can do to improve its condition and overall look.

happy and healthy

One of the many reasons I love to exercise and lead a healthy lifestyle is because it makes me feel fantastic. Working out with your buddies is naturally a real mood lifter and I can feel really zingy for hours after exercise.

I find working out a real stress-buster; if I'm worrying about something or I have a to-do list from hell, there's nothing like a bit of exercise to calm the mind. Sometimes, if you're going over that same niggling worry, a really good workout and stretch afterwards will get you back to an even keel.

Evidence shows that exercise releases endorphins – chemicals that trigger happy and positive feelings in the brain. These little fellas induce a feeling of euphoria after a really good workout. Exercise is commonly known to combat feelings of depression and low self-esteem, and interaction with people and emotional support is also crucial for a happy existence. So . . . exercise PLUS endorphins PLUS your buddies really does make for a winning formula!

Saying that, there are a few extra things I do to help me to relax and stay (relatively) sane in the hectic world that we all live in.

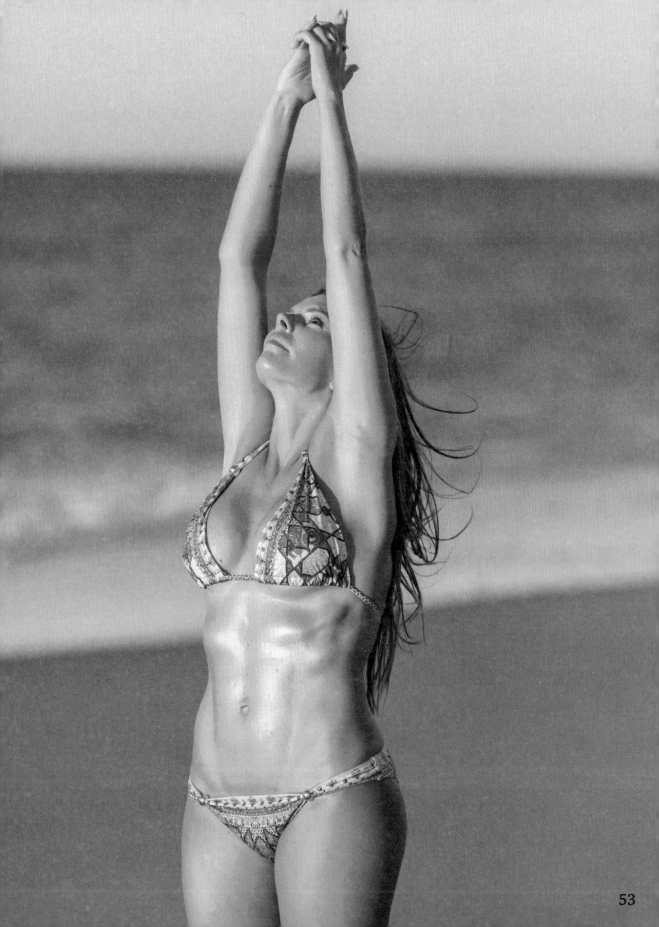

53

Whilst I love being with friends and family, I do like a bit of me time and I usually like to have at least half an hour a day on my own.

SLEEP

This is really important for me. Everyone feels so much happier, brighter and energetic after a good night's sleep and I'm certainly no exception. To wind down after a busy day, I'm pretty strict about switching off all electrical devices by 9.30pm, and I find reading puts me in the right mood for sleep. A bath with lavender salts is also really soothing, and great for any minor aches from a hard workout.

ME TIME

Whilst I love being with friends and family, I do like a bit of me time and I usually like to have at least half an hour a day on my own. I'll often take the dogs for a walk, just enjoying the moment, taking in the trees and sounds around me and trying not to think too much. I do like to keep moving, even very gently, so I'll often do a bit of stretching in front of the TV or in the garden. I find it relaxing, it's good for my back and improves flexibility all round.

FIND YOUR THING

All of us have that 'thing' that helps us unwind. It might be dog-walking, singing or splashing in puddles – whatever it is, do it if it makes you happy. I find riding horses incredibly calming and I know being with animals is the cure for many people's ills. I also love to do Pilates, particularly for my back, as it involves lots of lovely stretches and I feel so much longer and leaner after a good session. Sometimes when I'm stretching I'll close my eyes, slow down my breathing and try to focus on my body and the stretches I'm doing. This really helps to still and calm my mind, and is sometimes just what I need after a hectic day with the family or a tough workout.

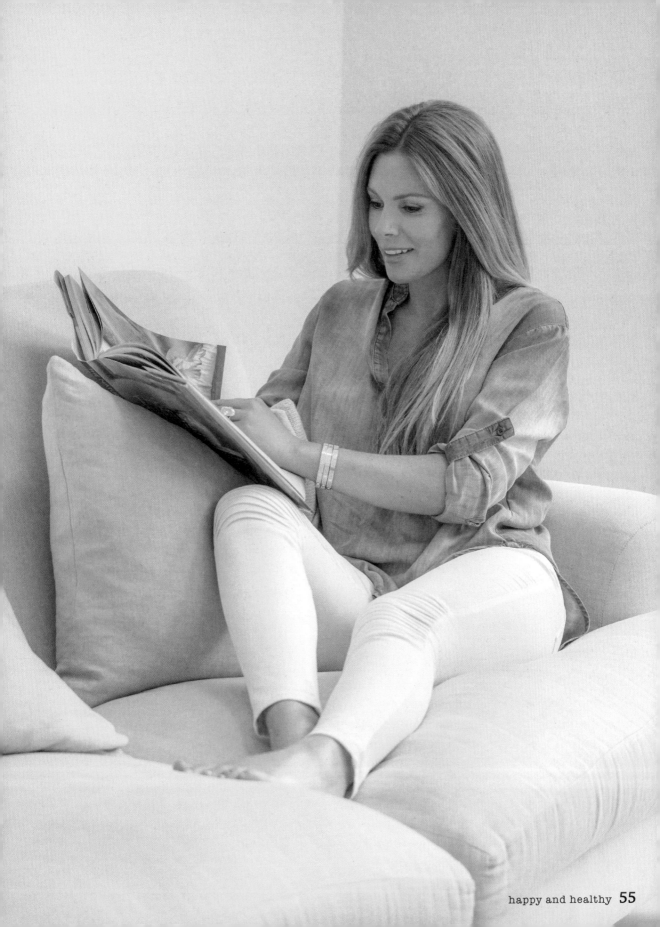

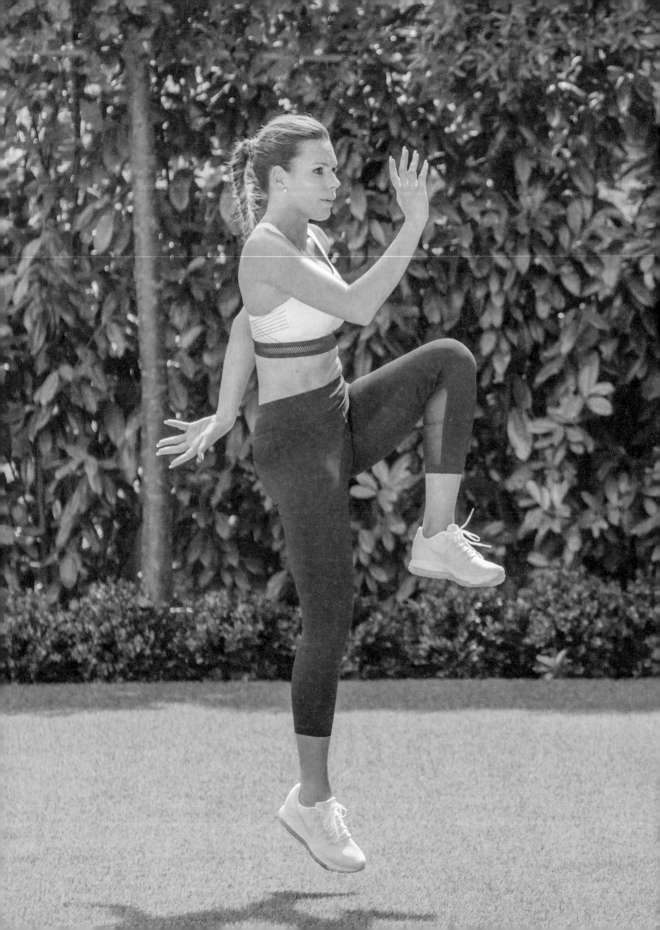

Now you need to get moving. Get out there, work hard and exercise with your buddies, family or on your own. It might be tough at first but keep at it and I promise you'll eventually feel stronger, leaner and happier. The key is to keep motivated, vary your workouts and have some fun! Combine this with eating well and you're well on the road to a healthy lifestyle.

train

So now your fitness journey begins. Hopefully you have all the inspiration you need to get going; all that is required now is some hard work. Everyone can do these exercises but you need a positive mindset to push yourself at every session and encourage those around you. Put the work in and you'll see the benefits after a few weeks – plus there really is nothing better than that post-workout buzz!

The exercises included in this book can all be done at home with the minimum of equipment and fuss. There are two specific partner workouts as well as exercises you can do with your buddies or on your own. I like to vary my workouts so I always do a combination of different types of workout. The workouts include warm-up and muscle activation exercises, partner workouts, HIIT workouts, cardio and circuit training and stretching exercises. All of these exercises form part of my weekly workout and you can select which exercises you want to do depending on your goals, experience and ability.

How you structure your programme is down to you and there's more information on this on page 162. Just as an example, I currently do two 30-minute HIIT workout sessions twice a week and one 60-minute circuit training session a week, either with buddies or on my own. I also combine this with activities with the family, a partner workout and stretching. Anyone new to exercise may choose to do two workouts a week and build from there – it's much better and safer for your body to start slowly. I wanted this book to be accessible as possible, so I've included exercises that are suitable for beginners as well as some more advanced options. As you progress, you can do more reps (repetitions – the number of times you do each exercise) or sets (a group of reps, after which you take a short rest). You can also do each exercise for longer and rest for a shorter time if doing a HIIT workout. If you're running, you can run further and faster, and if circuit training, as well as increasing your reps and sets, you can use heavier forms of equipment (see page 60).

As you train, however, make sure you listen to your body. Always warm up, activate your muscles, cool down, stretch and try to follow the exercises correctly. It's far better to keep your movements controlled and fluid rather than rush through them without paying any attention to the techniques. If you have any injuries, experience sharp pains or find any exercises particularly difficult, stop and seek advice from a health professional. Any injury will only set you back in your fitness journey, and your aim is to feel stronger and fitter, not the opposite!

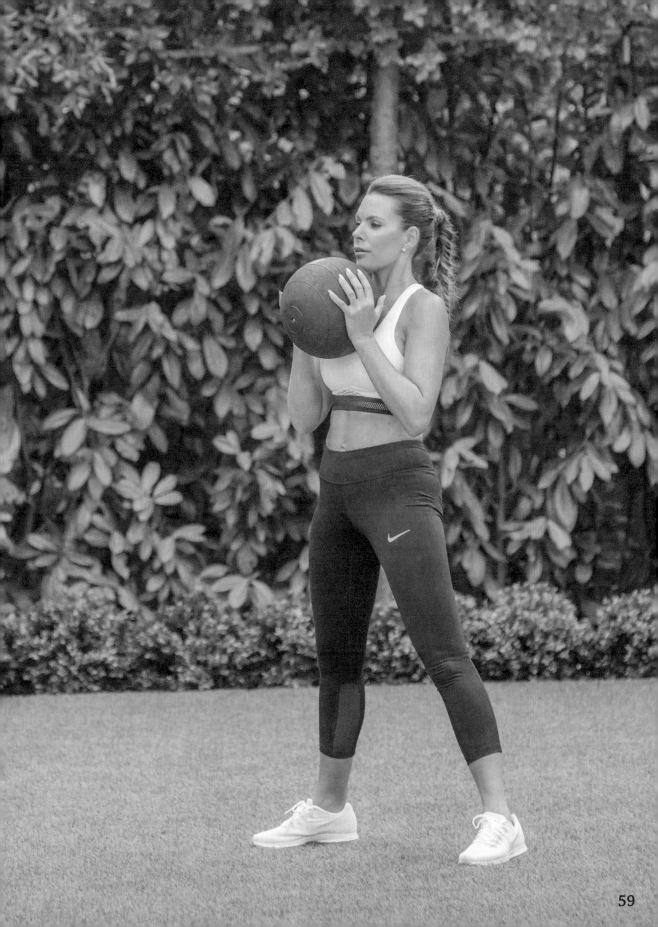

equipment

You'll need very little equipment for these exercises. Most require just your own or your buddy's body weight and a lot of gritty determination! For HIIT, circuit training and LISS cardio workouts, there are various apps you can download that will help you keep time during work and rest periods (see page 256). There is the odd exercise where a skipping rope or glute activation band is handy, and there are various items required for circuit training. Here's the lowdown on what's needed.

Battle rope – these thick, heavy ropes work every muscle group from arms and shoulders to abs and legs, all in one go. They are available on the web and in most gyms.

Resistance bands – these are very simple looped resistance bands that you can purchase on the internet or at retailers for very little money. They come in various sizes and widths for different resistance levels and to suit different body shapes and weight. These bands are great for glute activation exercises and do wonders for firming up that booty!

Skipping rope – you may well have one kicking around the house. If not, get yourself a lightweight skipping rope, adjust it to the correct length, and go skip!

Slam ball – a rubber, non-bouncing, dead weight of a ball which is perfect for resistance training. They range in weight from 2 to 20 kg, depending on your ability and strength.

Weights – Buy yourself a couple of weights – lower weight ones to begin with and then move on to heavier ones as you progress. Beginners might like to try something between 2 and 4 kilograms. You should be able to perform 10 reps without losing your technique. If you find the exercise easy, then move on to something a little heavier.

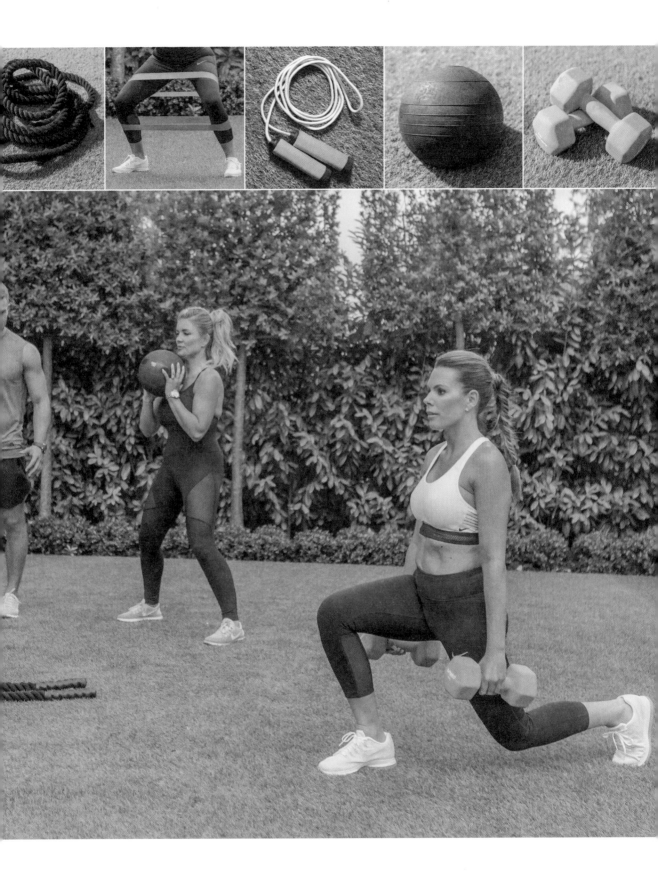

fitness terms

There are lots of technical words and terms bandied about when it comes to fitness. For those who work in the industry, it's obvious what they all mean. For everyone else, it's sometimes useful to have a bit of clarification! Here's what some of the more common words and expressions mean.

CARDIOVASCULAR

Relates to the heart and blood vessels. Cardiovascular fitness or exercise (cardio for short) gets your heart rate up and delivers oxygen to your muscles. A strong cardiovascular system helps the heart to pump blood and oxygen around the body, equips the body to burn fat cells, builds muscle tone and improves overall health.

CIRCUIT TRAINING

Involves short bursts of resistance training, often using moderate weights and equipment. Circuit training improves strength, tones the muscles and burns fat at the same time.

CORE

Core muscles are found in the pelvis, lower back, abdomen and hips. A strong core stabilizes the body, protects the spinal column and provides a strong support for all sorts of physical activity. When you engage or strengthen your core, you contract the deepest abdominal muscles. To find these muscles place your hands on the bony parts of the front of your hips, then move them an inch towards your belly button and an inch down. Contract the muscles by drawing your navel in towards your spine and keep them contracted by about 30 per cent during an exercise.

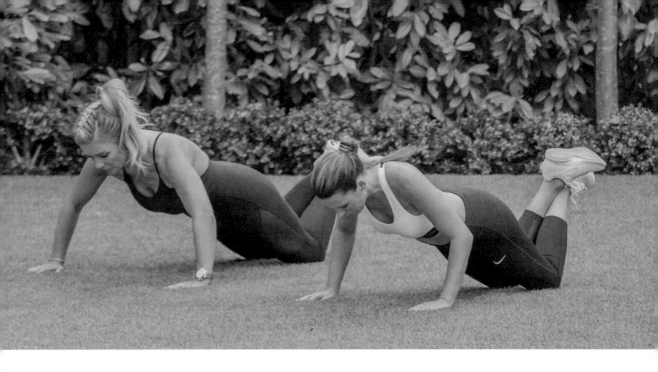

GLUTES
A group of three muscles that make up your bottom!

HAMSTRING
Tendons behind your knee that join the muscles of your thigh to the bones of your lower leg.

HIIT
Short for high-intensity interval training, this is a cardiovascular exercise that involves short periods of intense exercise followed by short periods of recovery.
This form of exercise gets the heart pumping, builds muscle, burns fat and improves endurance.

LISS
Short for low-intensity steady state. It's a lower intensity cardio workout performed over a longer, continuous period and puts less stress on the body. Walking, jogging and cycling are all examples of LISS training.

LUMBAR
The lumbar muscles are those found in the lower back, known as the lumbar spine.

QUADS
Short for quadriceps, these make up the large muscle at the front of the thigh.

REPS
Short for repetitions, the number of times you do each exercise.

SETS
A group of repetitions of an exercise, after which you take a short rest.

warming up

Warming up before you work out is an important part of any exercise programme. A good warm-up should gradually increase your heart rate, boost circulation to your muscles and mentally prepare you for a workout. Warming up your muscles, tendons and ligaments minimises the risk of injury. I warm up for around 10–15 minutes either with a gentle jog or skip, or some body-weight warm-ups and a quick glute activation session.

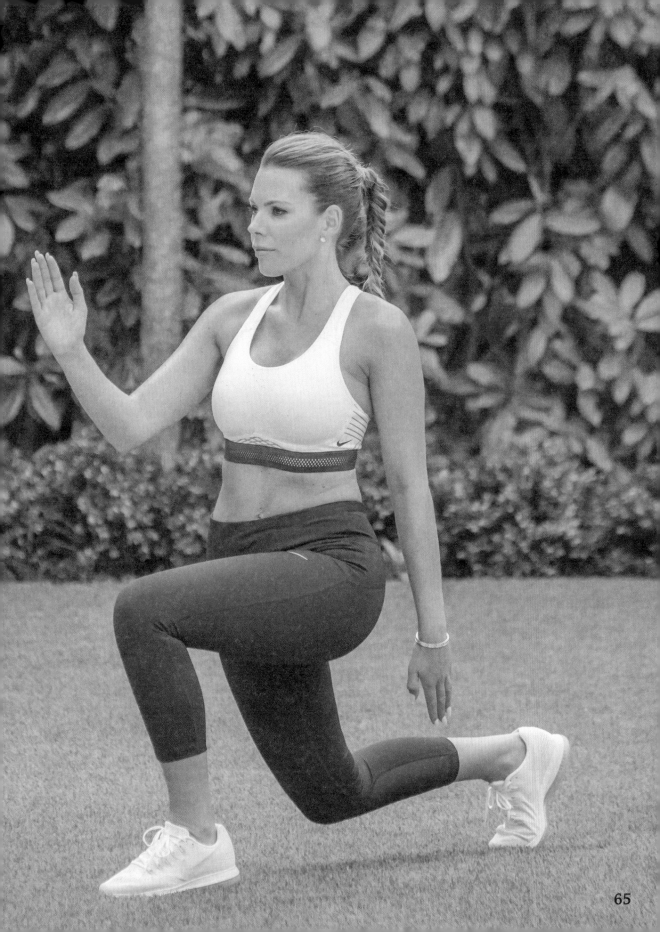

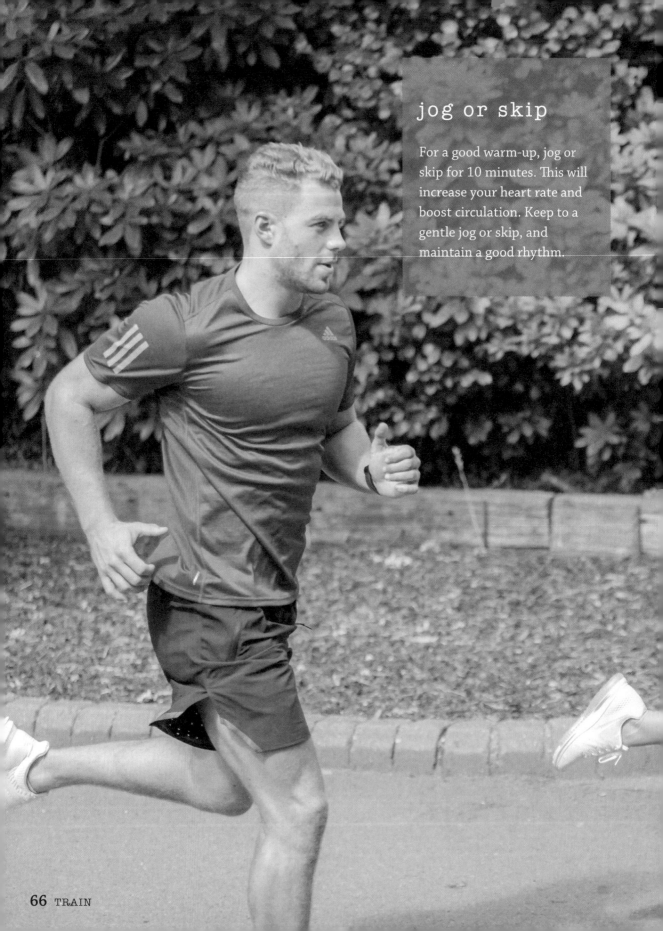

jog or skip

For a good warm-up, jog or skip for 10 minutes. This will increase your heart rate and boost circulation. Keep to a gentle jog or skip, and maintain a good rhythm.

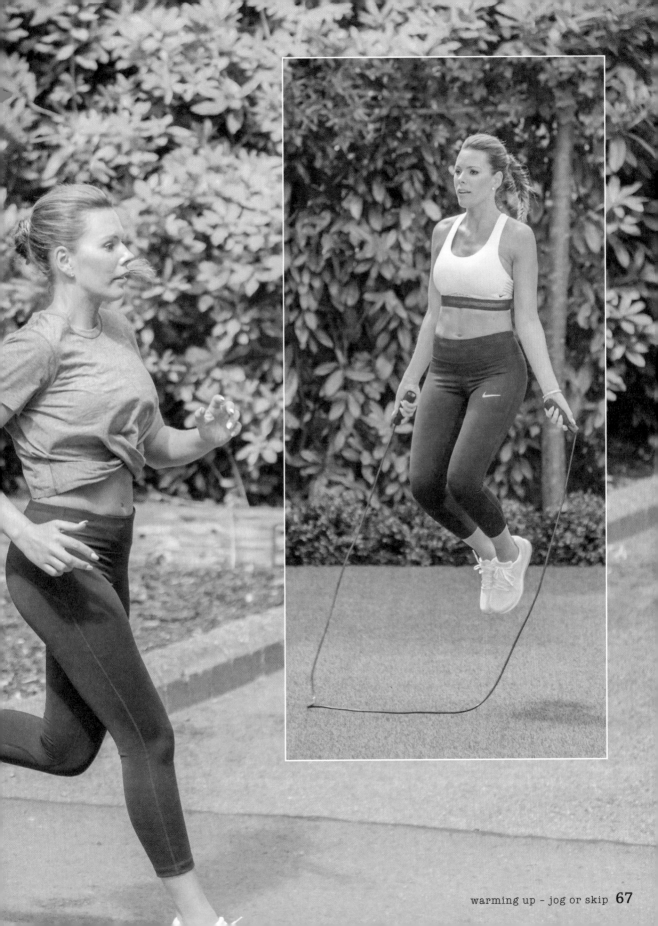

glute activation

Before working out it's a good idea to 'switch on' those glute muscles, especially if you're going to be doing lots of lower-body exercises. This ensures the correct muscles are working when you exercise. Do this exercise for 40 seconds, then rest for 20 seconds, and repeat three times.

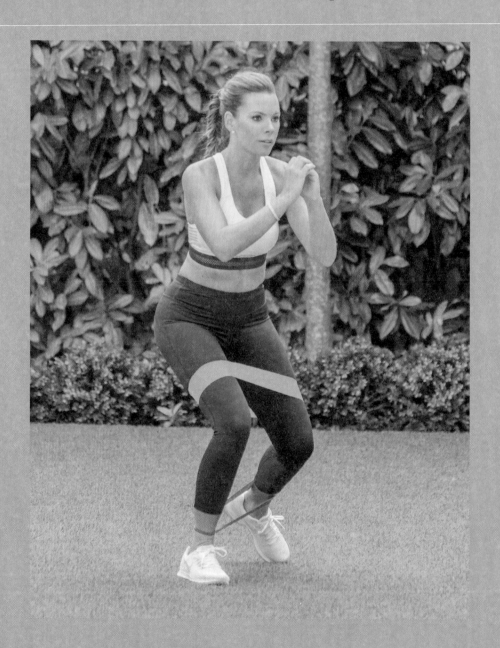

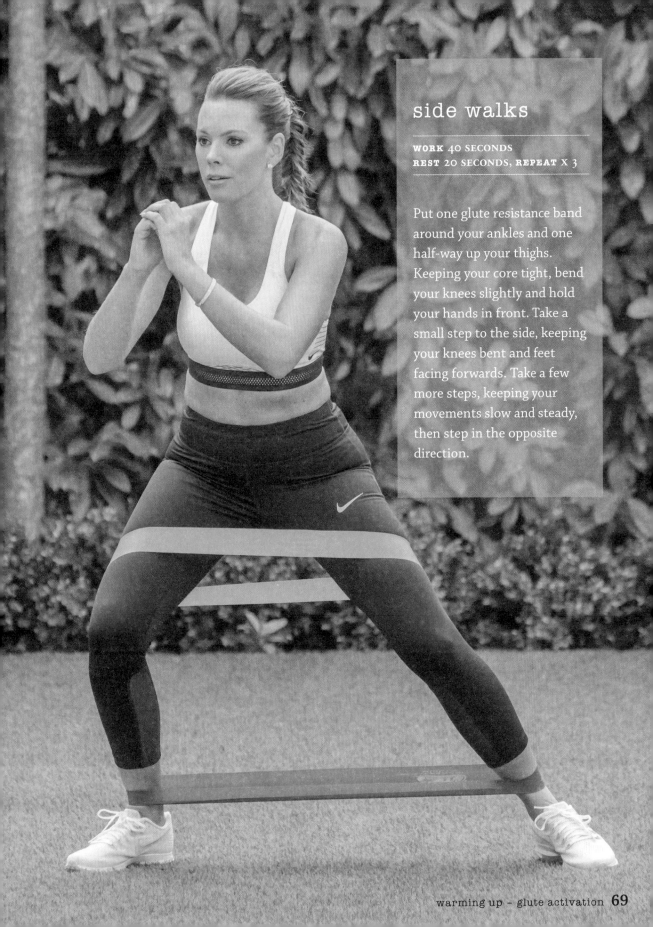

side walks

WORK 40 SECONDS
REST 20 SECONDS, **REPEAT** X 3

Put one glute resistance band around your ankles and one half-way up your thighs. Keeping your core tight, bend your knees slightly and hold your hands in front. Take a small step to the side, keeping your knees bent and feet facing forwards. Take a few more steps, keeping your movements slow and steady, then step in the opposite direction.

body-weight warm-ups

These set of exercises provide an alternative 15-minute warm-up. They use the body weight as resistance and help to warm up the muscles and increase your heart rate. Do each exercise for 40 seconds, then rest for 20 seconds and repeat three times.

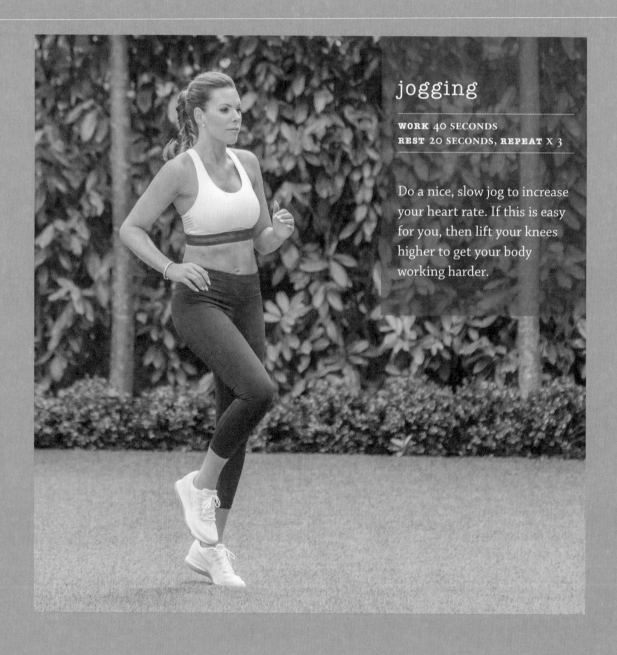

jogging

WORK 40 SECONDS
REST 20 SECONDS, **REPEAT** X 3

Do a nice, slow jog to increase your heart rate. If this is easy for you, then lift your knees higher to get your body working harder.

star jumps

WORK 40 SECONDS
REST 20 SECONDS, **REPEAT** X 3

1 Stand, with your arms down.

2 Lift your arms and jump into a star position, keeping your arms and legs straight and core engaged. Return to the original standing position.

ADVANCED Start from a squat position, toes pointing outwards, heels down and straight arms in front with hands together. As you jump up, throw your arms upwards. Return to the squat position.

ADVANCED

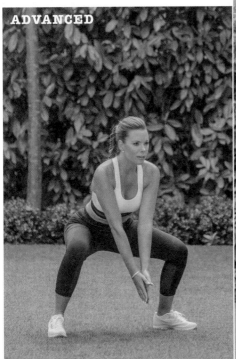

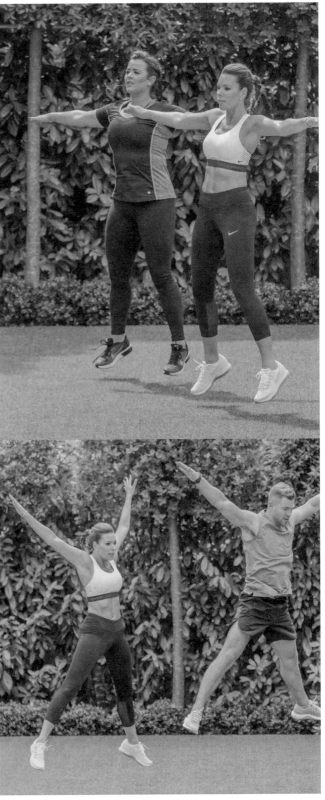

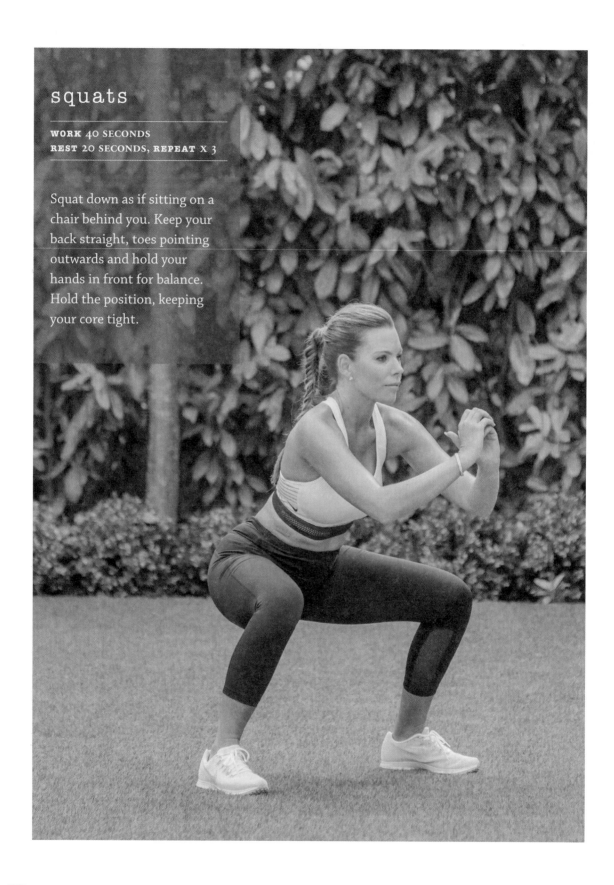

squats

WORK 40 SECONDS
REST 20 SECONDS, **REPEAT** X 3

Squat down as if sitting on a
chair behind you. Keep your
back straight, toes pointing
outwards and hold your
hands in front for balance.
Hold the position, keeping
your core tight.

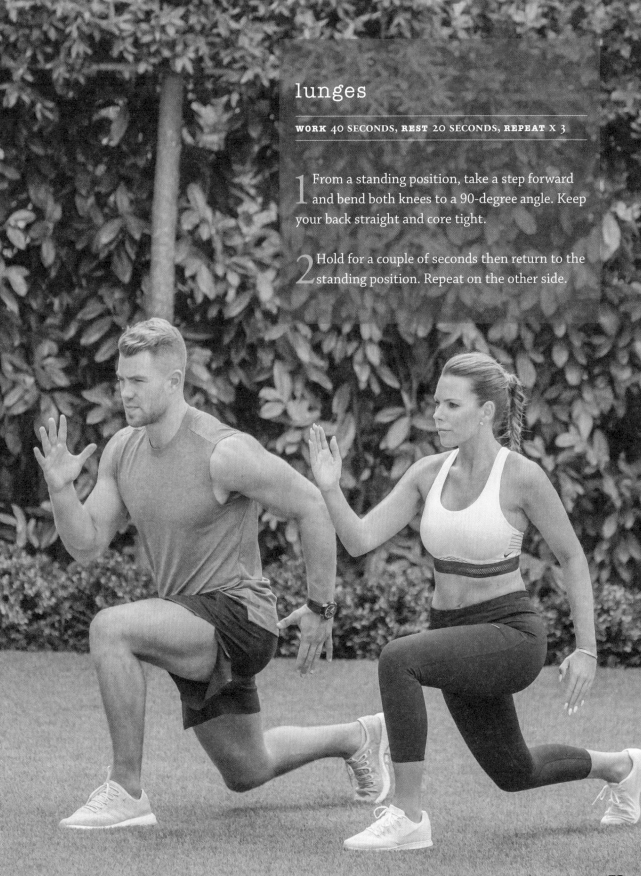

lunges

WORK 40 SECONDS, **REST** 20 SECONDS, **REPEAT** x 3

1 From a standing position, take a step forward and bend both knees to a 90-degree angle. Keep your back straight and core tight.

2 Hold for a couple of seconds then return to the standing position. Repeat on the other side.

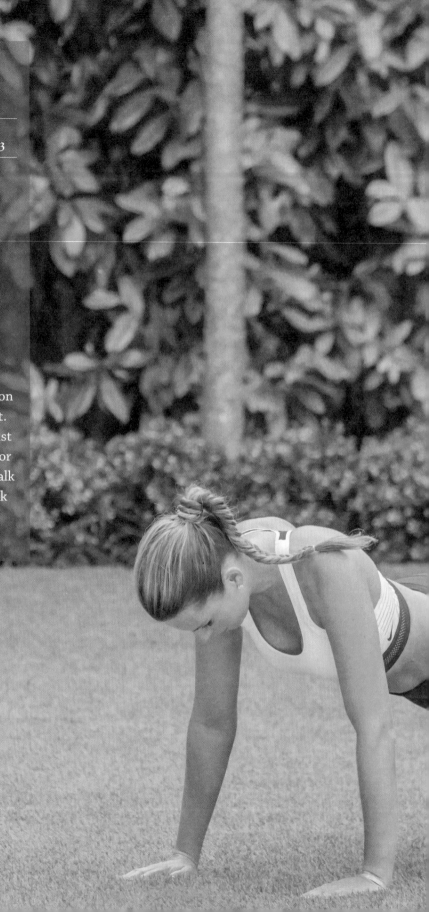

core walkouts

WORK 40 SECONDS
REST 20 SECONDS, **REPEAT** X 3

1 Start in a plank position, with core engaged, body straight, head aligned and hands under the shoulders.

2 Walk your hands back towards your feet.

3 Continue walking your hands back into an A position, with your heels on the ground and legs straight. (If you can't manage this, just do the best you can.) Hold for a couple of seconds, then walk your hands back to the plank position, and repeat.

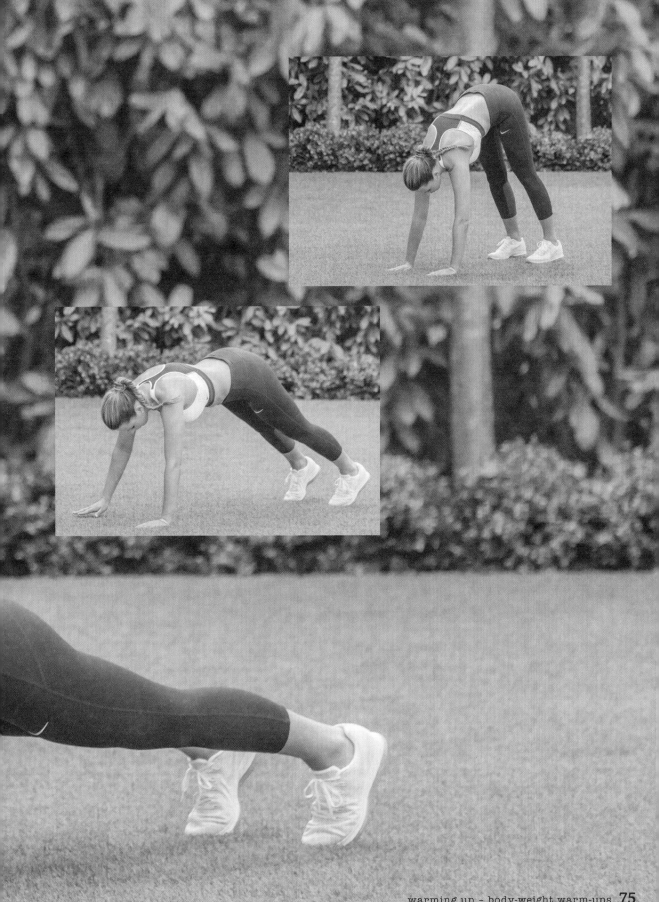

partner workouts

These two workouts are aimed specifically at partners working out together. Each workout includes six exercises and maximum effort is required! You should aim to do each exercise for 40 seconds, followed by 20 seconds of rest. Move on to the next exercise and complete five rounds of the exercises.

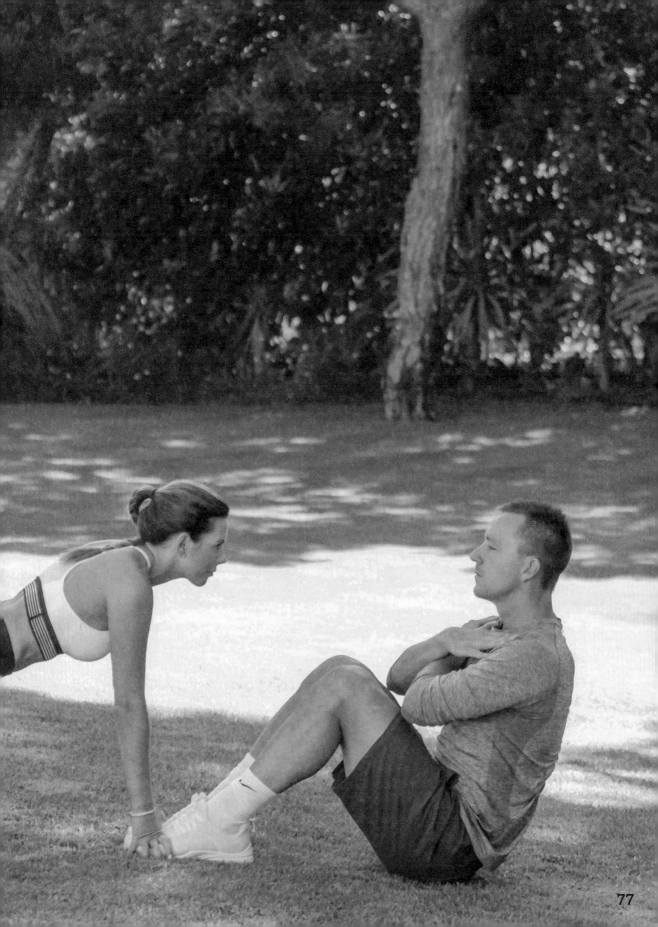

partner workout 1

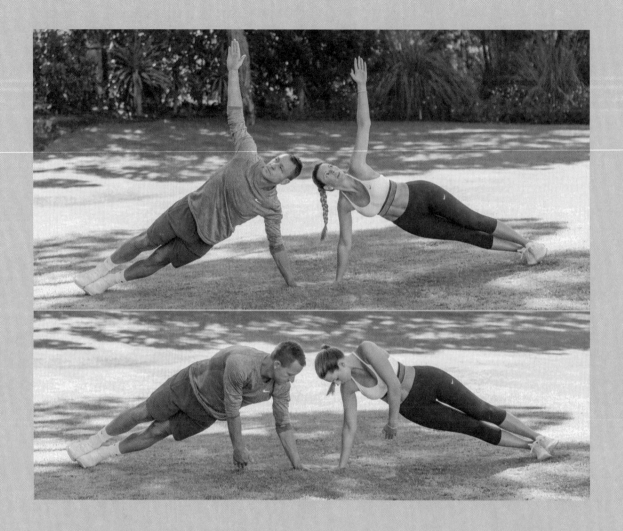

side plank with rotation

WORK 40 SECONDS, **REST** 20 SECONDS

1 You and your partner lie on your sides. Straighten your lower arm and lift your body, raising your upper arm. Keep your body straight and core strong.

2 Bring the upper arm down and across the body, following it with your eyes. Raise it up again and repeat.

squat jumps

WORK 40 SECONDS, **REST** 20 SECONDS

1 Start in a squat position, knees bent, core engaged and hands in front of you.

2 Jump up, throwing your arms down, and return to the squat position. Repeat.

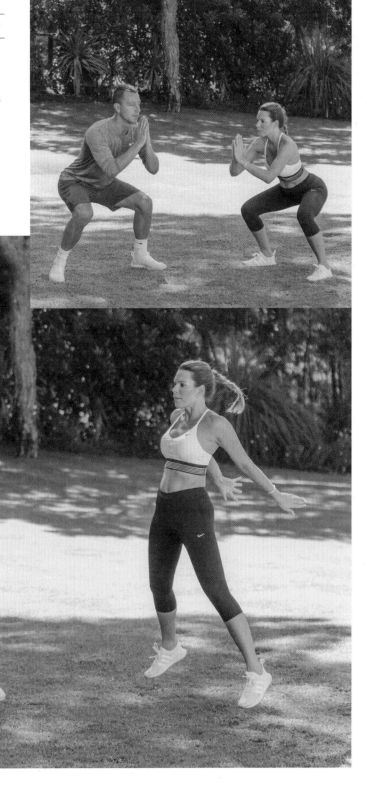

plank and crunch

WORK 40 SECONDS, **REST** 20 SECONDS

1 Your partner begins on their back in a sit-up position, knees bent and hands either side of their head. You start in a plank position, keeping a straight line from your shoulders to toes and core engaged, with your hands on your partner's feet.

2 Your partner lifts their upper body, arms still up by their head and core engaged, then returns to the starting position. They repeat while you maintain the plank position. After the first set, swap positions with you doing sit-ups and your partner in the plank position.

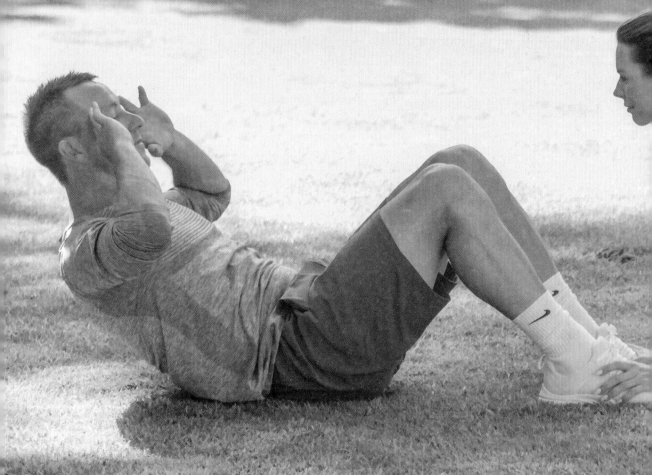

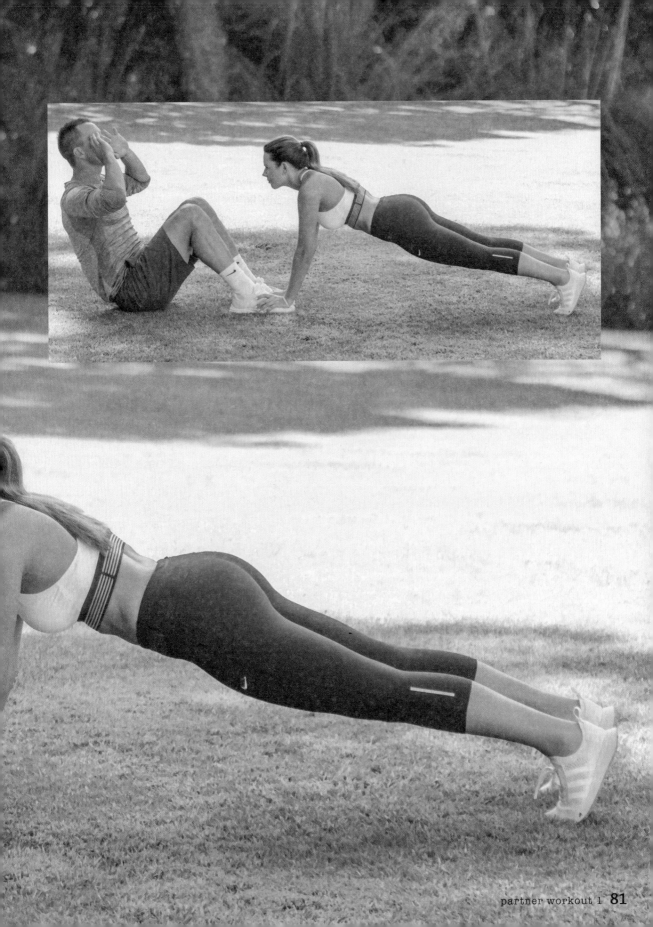

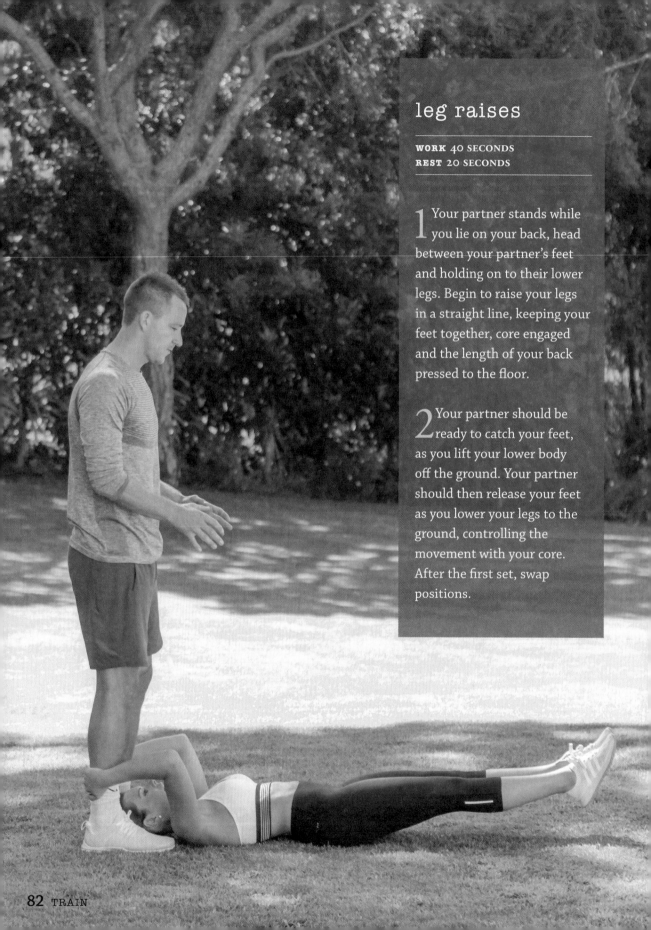

leg raises

WORK 40 SECONDS
REST 20 SECONDS

1 Your partner stands while you lie on your back, head between your partner's feet and holding on to their lower legs. Begin to raise your legs in a straight line, keeping your feet together, core engaged and the length of your back pressed to the floor.

2 Your partner should be ready to catch your feet, as you lift your lower body off the ground. Your partner should then release your feet as you lower your legs to the ground, controlling the movement with your core. After the first set, swap positions.

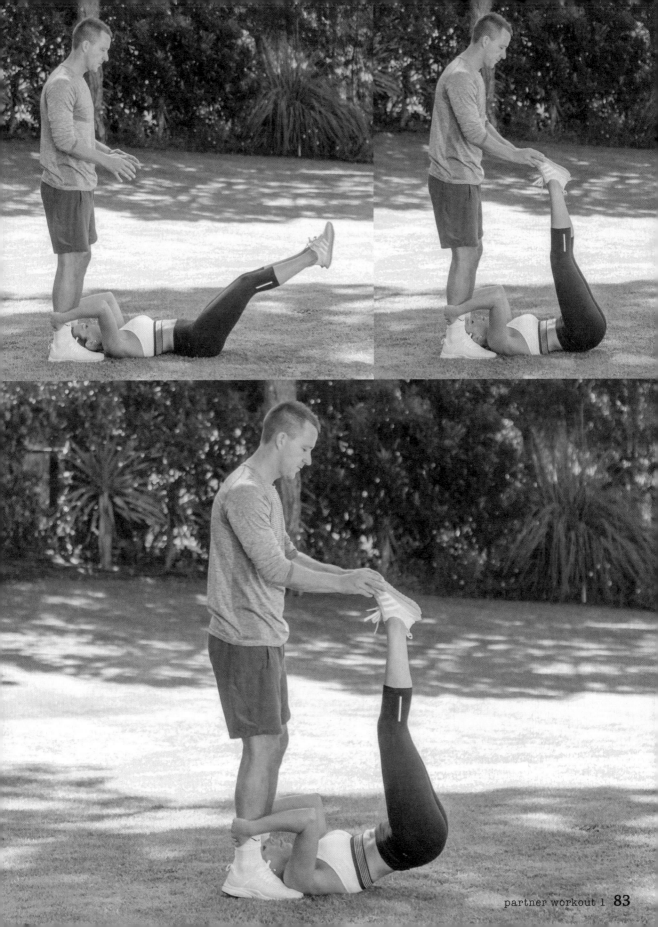

around the world

1 Sit on the ground facing your partner with your legs stretched out, feet slightly overlapping. Lean back, bend your elbows and lift your legs off the ground, keeping your legs straight, core engaged and without arching your back.

2 Circle your feet around your partner's feet as they rotate their legs in the opposite direction. Then change direction, keeping your core strong throughout.

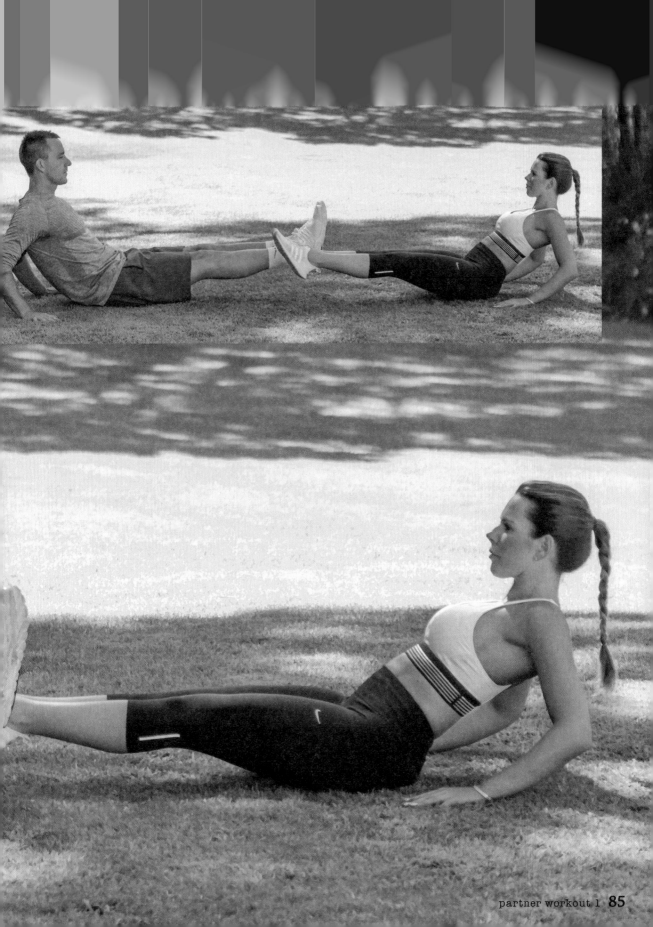

lunge knee-ups

WORK 40 SECONDS, **REST** 20 SECONDS

1 Step forward into a lunge position, with knees bent at 90 degrees.

2 Straighten the front leg and bring the back leg up to the front, keeping
the knee bent at 90 degrees. Return to the lunge position and repeat,
switching legs each time.

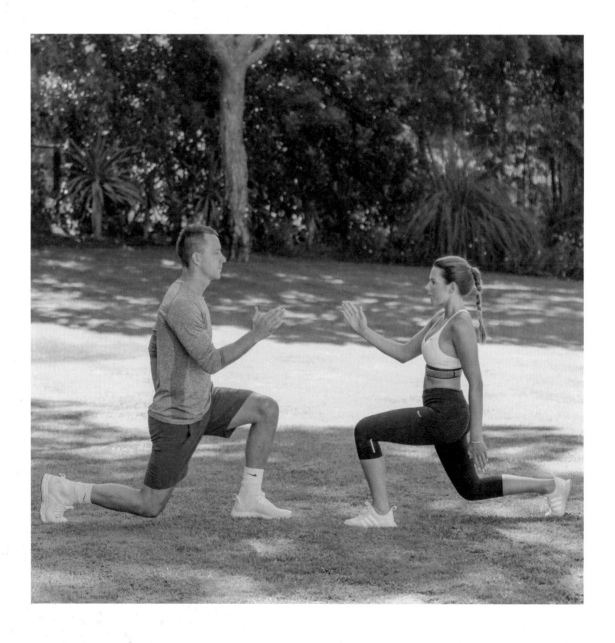

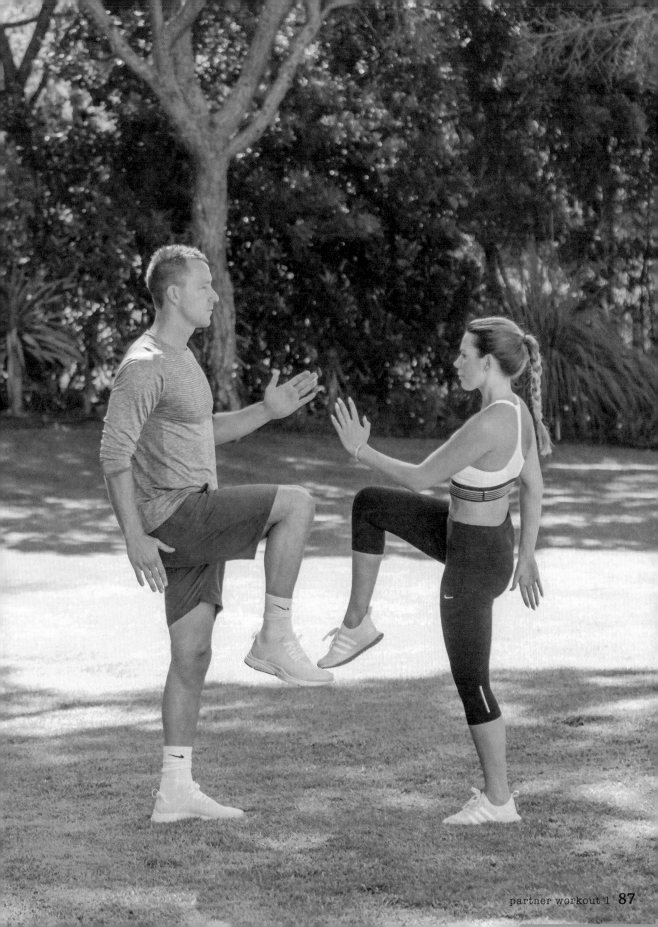

partner workout 2

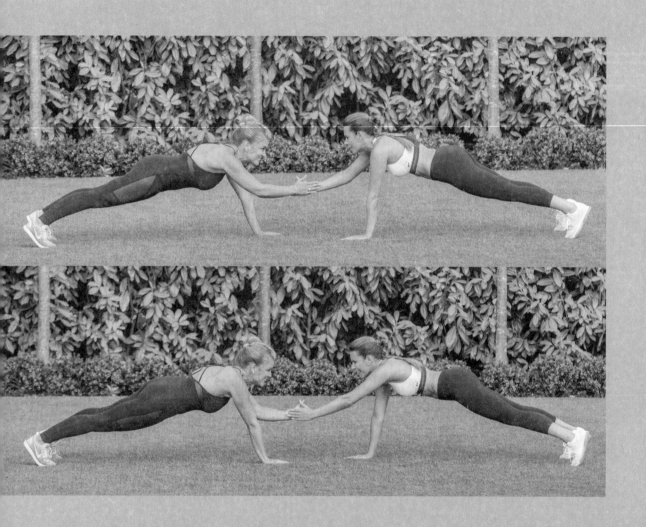

plank with claps

WORK 40 SECONDS, **REST** 20 SECONDS

1 Start in a plank position facing your partner, feet and arms hip-width apart, toes tucked under and body in a straight line. Engage your core.

2 Reach forward with one arm to clap your partner's opposite hand. Return to the starting position and repeat with the opposite arm.

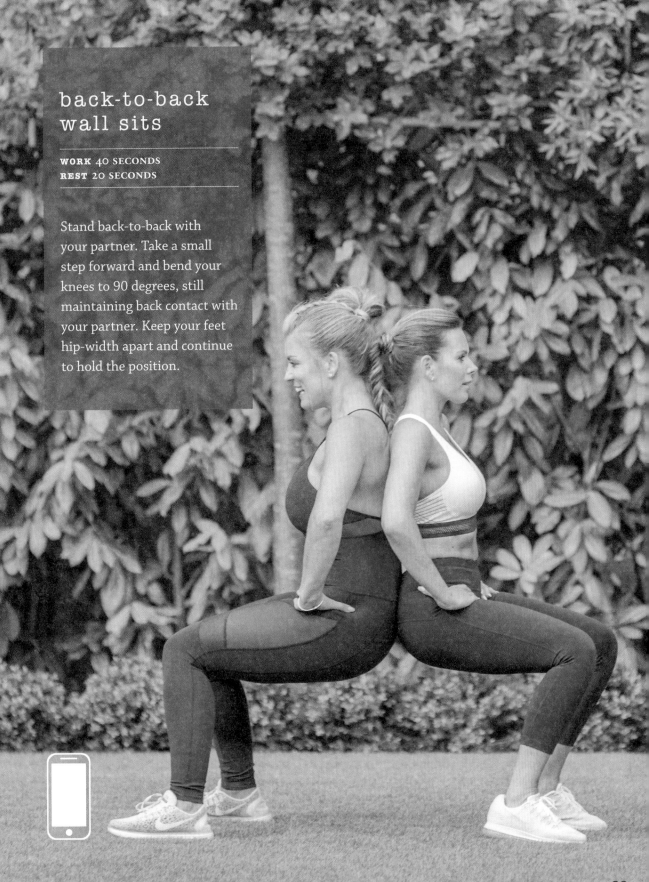

back-to-back
wall sits

WORK 40 SECONDS
REST 20 SECONDS

Stand back-to-back with
your partner. Take a small
step forward and bend your
knees to 90 degrees, still
maintaining back contact with
your partner. Keep your feet
hip-width apart and continue
to hold the position.

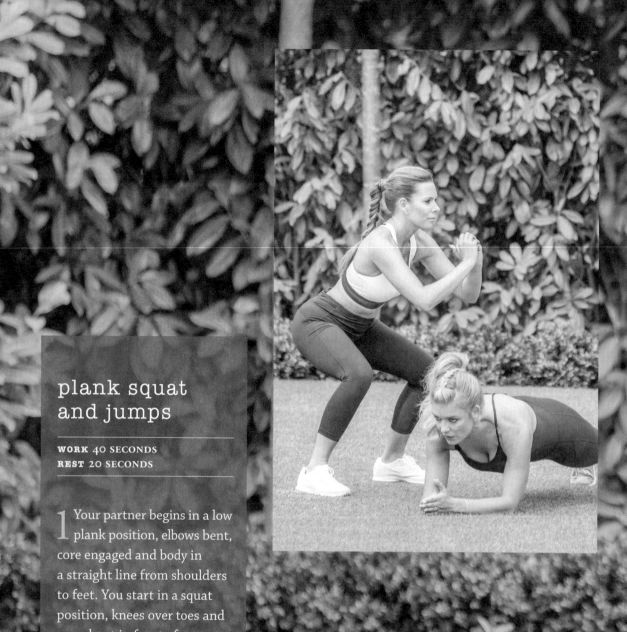

plank squat and jumps

WORK 40 SECONDS
REST 20 SECONDS

1 Your partner begins in a low plank position, elbows bent, core engaged and body in a straight line from shoulders to feet. You start in a squat position, knees over toes and arms bent in front of you.

2 As your partner maintains their plank position, you jump over them, landing in a squat position on the other side. Repeat and after one set swap positions with your partner.

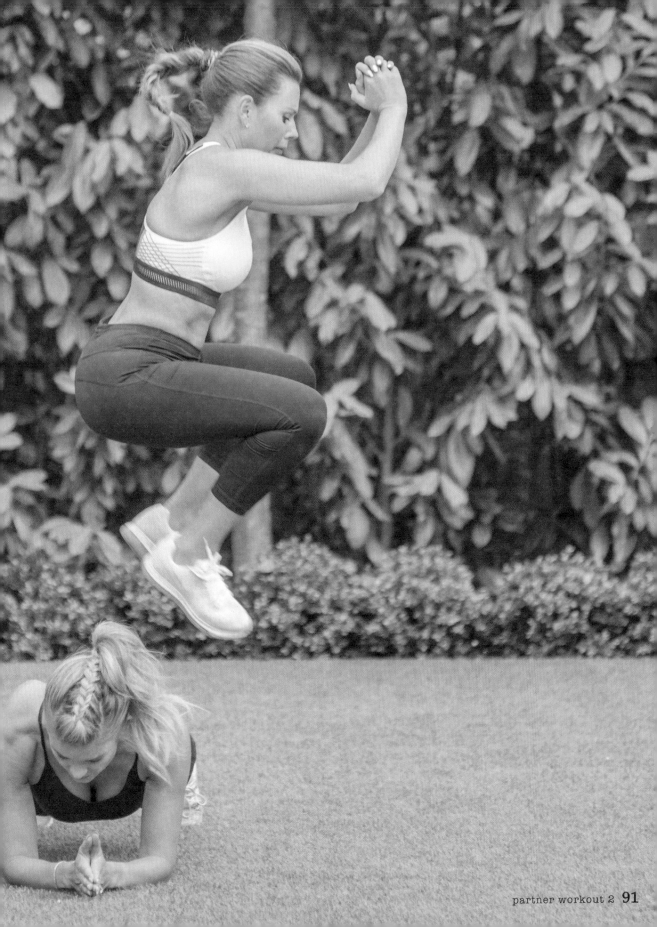

crunch and clap

1 Lie on the ground with your knees bent and hands either side of your head. Your partner stands with their toes overlapping yours, ready to clap your hands.

2 Lift your upper body until you can clap your partner's hands. Slowly lower your back to the ground, keeping your core engaged throughout. Repeat for a full set, then swap positions with your partner.

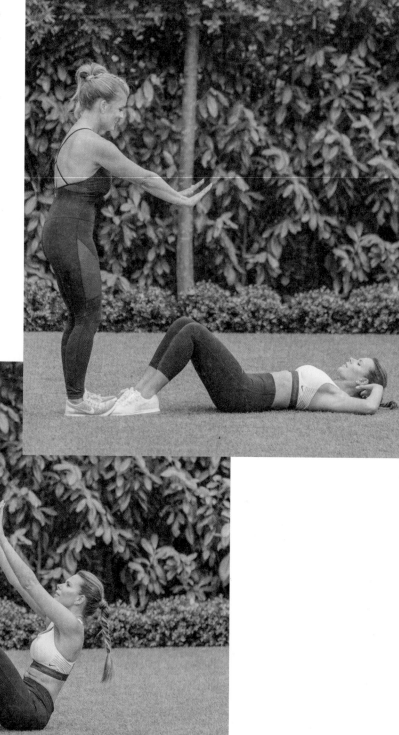

squat and
leg raise

WORK 40 SECONDS, **REST** 20 SECONDS

1 Stand with your feet by your partner's head as they lie on their back with legs raised. Hold on to their feet.

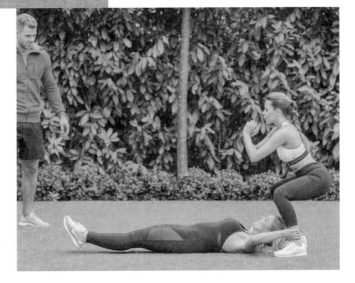

2 Let go of your partner's feet whilst they begin to lower their legs, keeping their core strong and back pressed to the ground. As they do this, bend your knees into a squat position.

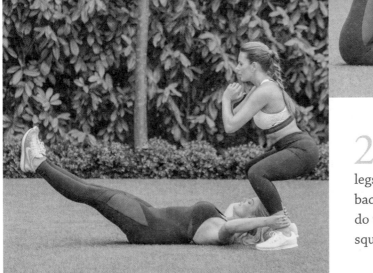

3 As your partner lowers their legs to the ground, you continue squatting as if sitting on a chair behind you. Your partner then raises their legs up as you straighten your knees and stand up. Repeat for a full set, then swap positions with your partner.

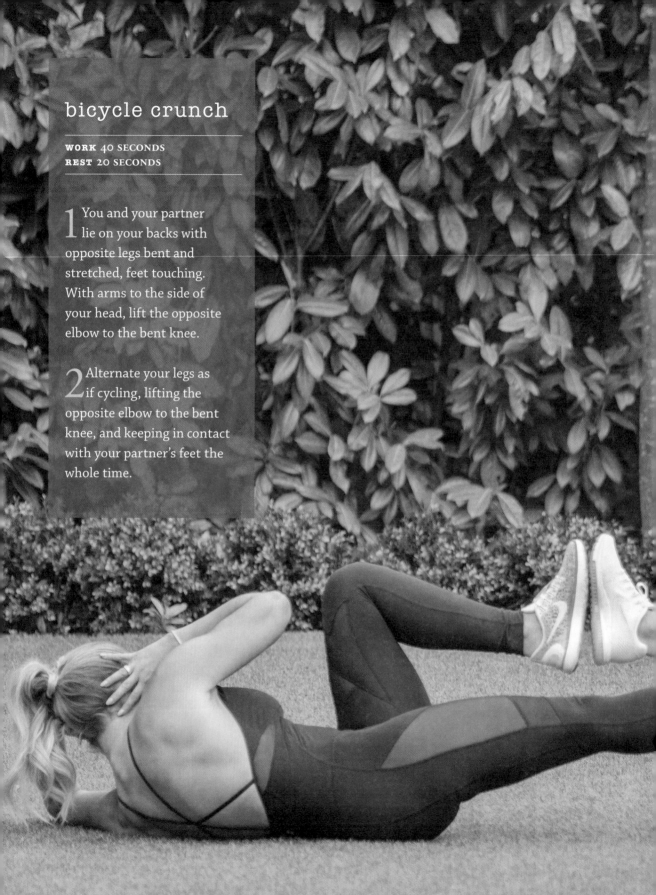

bicycle crunch

WORK 40 SECONDS
REST 20 SECONDS

1 You and your partner lie on your backs with opposite legs bent and stretched, feet touching. With arms to the side of your head, lift the opposite elbow to the bent knee.

2 Alternate your legs as if cycling, lifting the opposite elbow to the bent knee, and keeping in contact with your partner's feet the whole time.

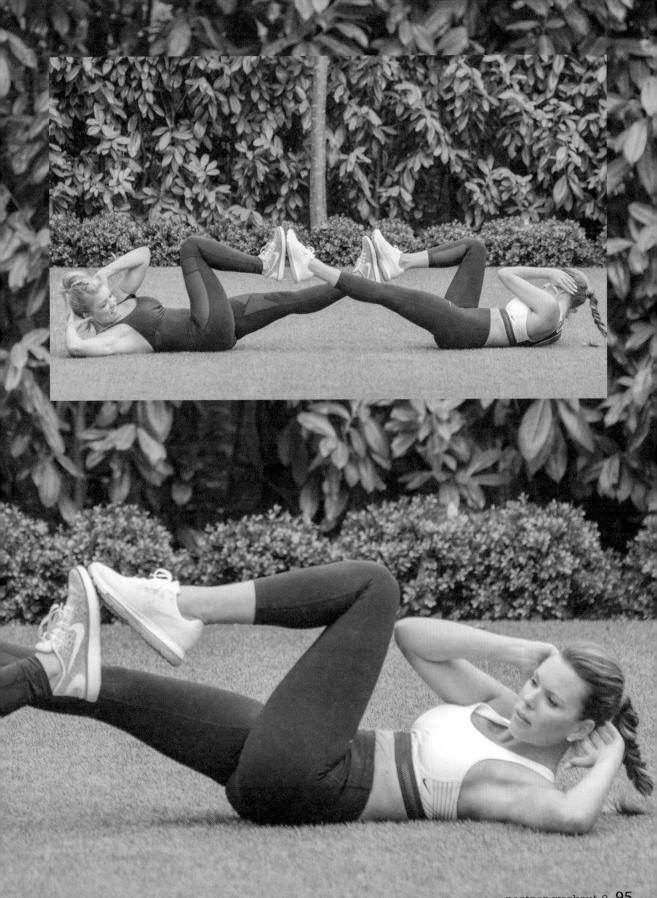

HIIT workouts

HIIT workouts – high-intensity interval training – are short and intense workouts. It's an incredibly efficient form of exercise and great for those who are short on time. A high-impact cardiovascular form of exercise, HIIT boosts endurance and gives your metabolism a real kickstart.

The exercises are divided into different sections, relating to the area of the body they work. The aim is to push yourself hard and to complete 30 seconds of each exercise, followed by 30 seconds of rest. (If you're more advanced, complete 40 seconds of each exercise, followed by 20 seconds of rest.) Move on to the next exercise, and then complete five rounds of each section.

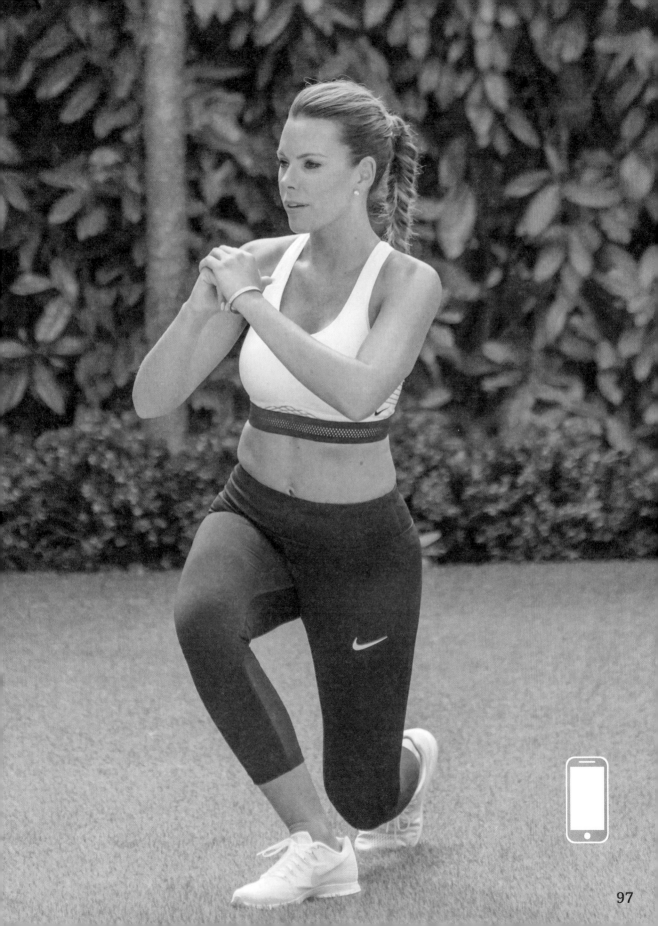

lower body

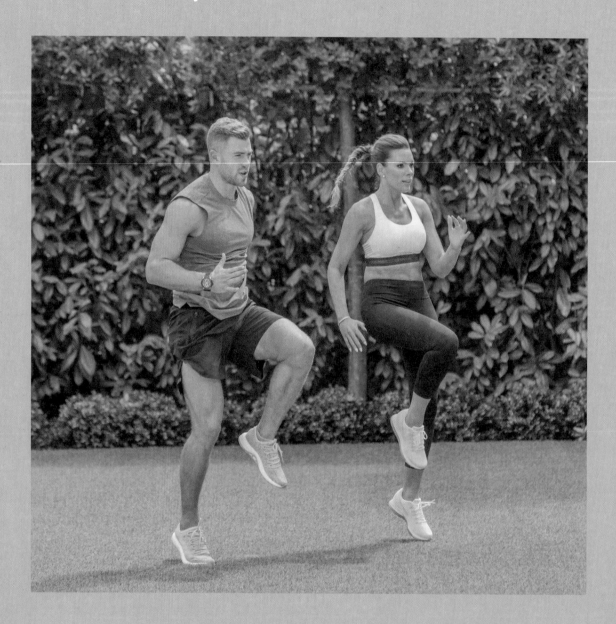

sprint on the spot

WORK 30 SECONDS, **REST** 30 SECONDS

Sprint on the spot, raising each knee high,
well above the knee of the other leg.

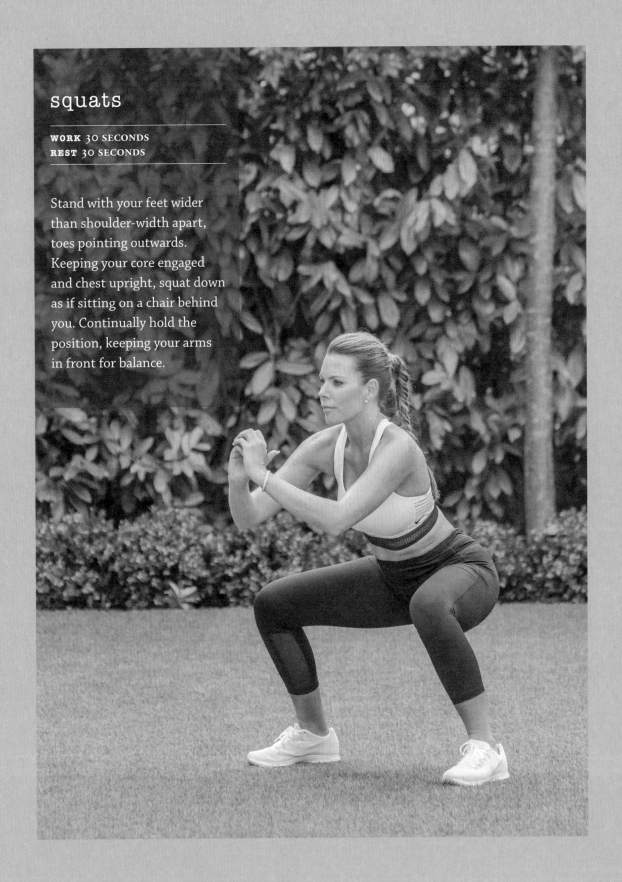

squats

WORK 30 SECONDS
REST 30 SECONDS

Stand with your feet wider
than shoulder-width apart,
toes pointing outwards.
Keeping your core engaged
and chest upright, squat down
as if sitting on a chair behind
you. Continually hold the
position, keeping your arms
in front for balance.

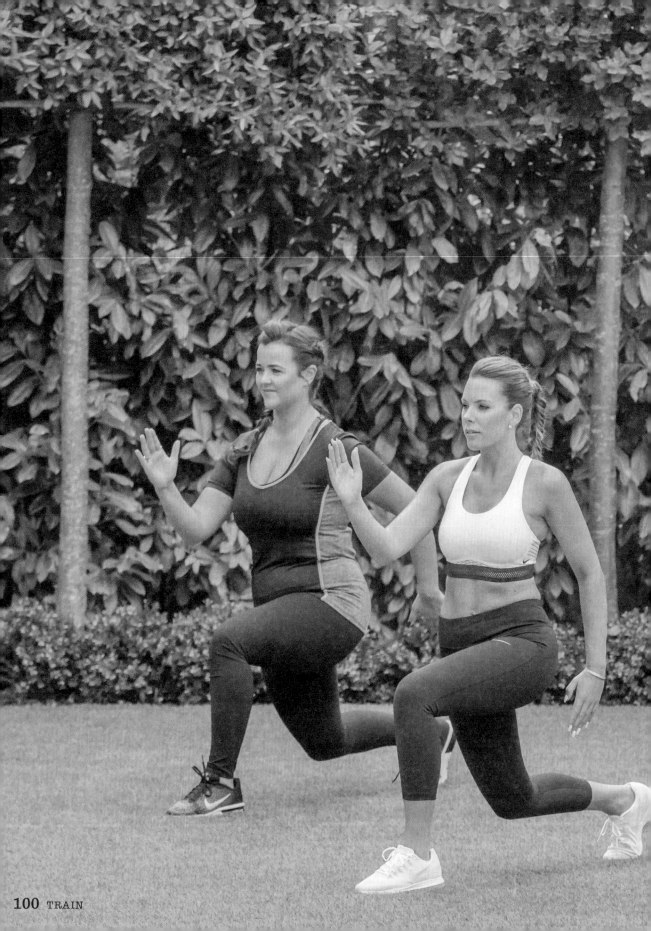

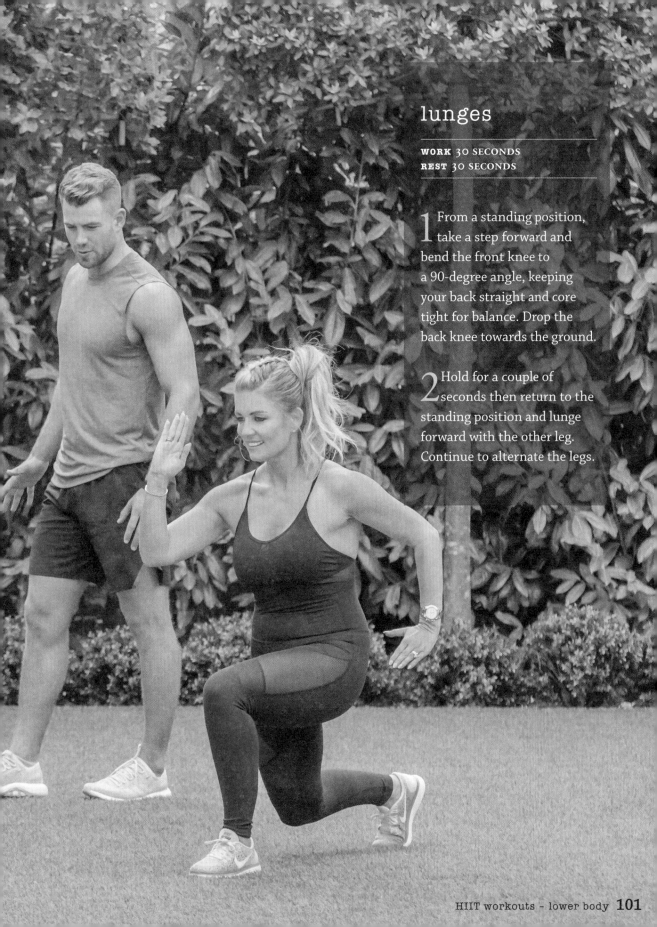

lunges

WORK 30 SECONDS
REST 30 SECONDS

1 From a standing position, take a step forward and bend the front knee to a 90-degree angle, keeping your back straight and core tight for balance. Drop the back knee towards the ground.

2 Hold for a couple of seconds then return to the standing position and lunge forward with the other leg. Continue to alternate the legs.

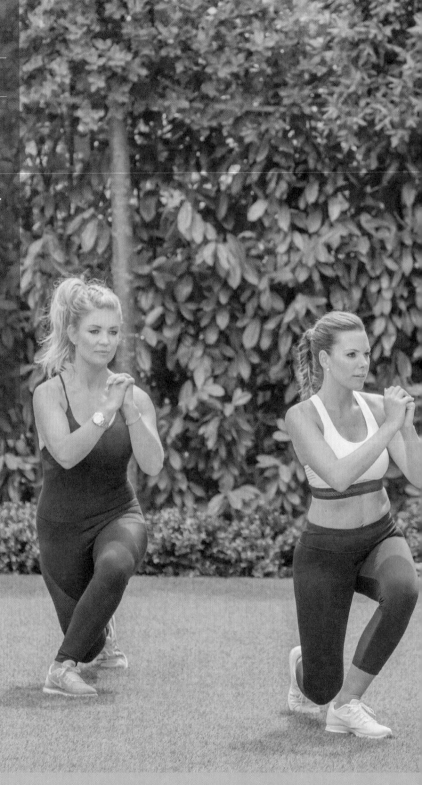

curtsy lunges

WORK 30 SECONDS
REST 30 SECONDS

1 Start from a standing position and step your left leg behind you and to the right so your thighs cross. Bend both knees as if you are curtsying. Keep your core tight, back straight and hold your hands in front for balance.

2 Hold for a couple of seconds, then return to the standing position and repeat on the other side.

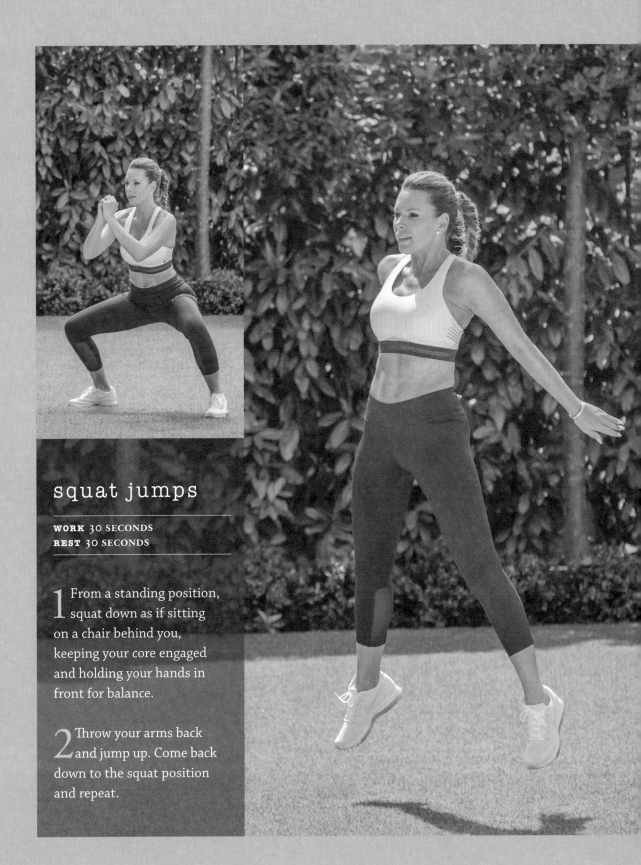

squat jumps

WORK 30 SECONDS
REST 30 SECONDS

1 From a standing position, squat down as if sitting on a chair behind you, keeping your core engaged and holding your hands in front for balance.

2 Throw your arms back and jump up. Come back down to the squat position and repeat.

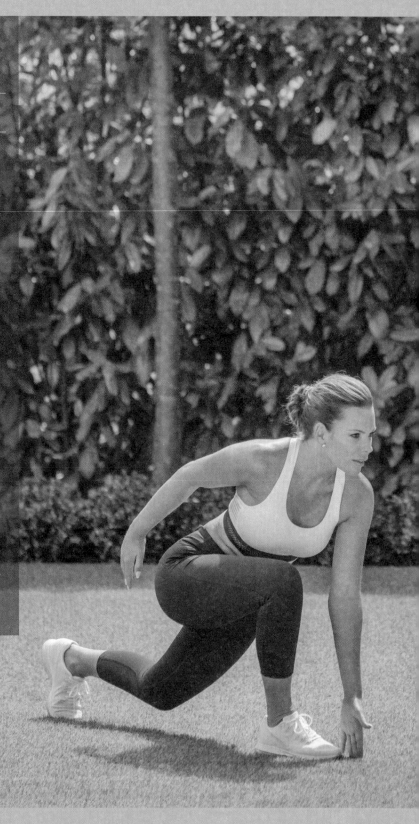

runner's lunge

WORK 30 SECONDS
REST 30 SECONDS

1 Standing with one foot in front of the other, drop down, bending your front knee to a 90-degree angle, knee above the toe.

2 Straighten the front leg, bring the back leg up in front and bend that knee to a 90-degree angle. Return to the original lunge position and repeat, keeping the movement controlled and the core engaged. After one set swap sides.

ADVANCED From the runner's lunge position, introduce a jump as you bring the back leg to the front, then return to the original lunge position. Repeat and swap sides.

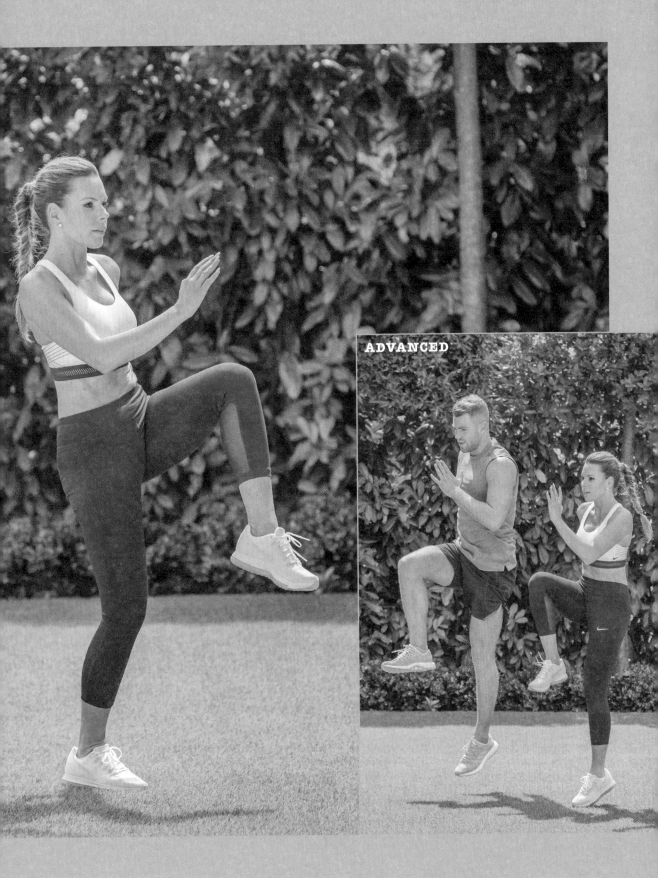

ADVANCED

upper body and core

plank

WORK 30 SECONDS
REST 30 SECONDS

Get into a low plank position with your body in a straight line, elbows bent and arms and feet shoulder-width apart. Keep your core tight and continue to hold the position.

ADVANCED In the plank position, rotate your body to one side and dip your hip almost to the floor. Return to the starting position, repeat on the other side and keep alternating sides.

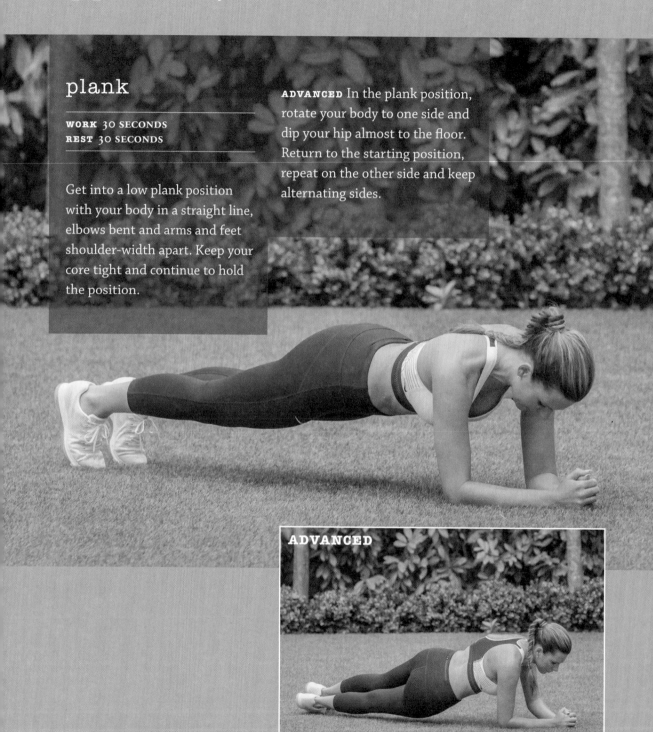

ADVANCED

up-down plank

WORK 30 SECONDS

REST 30 SECONDS

1 Start in a low plank position. Engage your core and tuck your feet under.

2 Straighten one arm and then the other, then bend each elbow and return to the low plank position. Repeat this up and down movement, alternating which arm you straighten first.

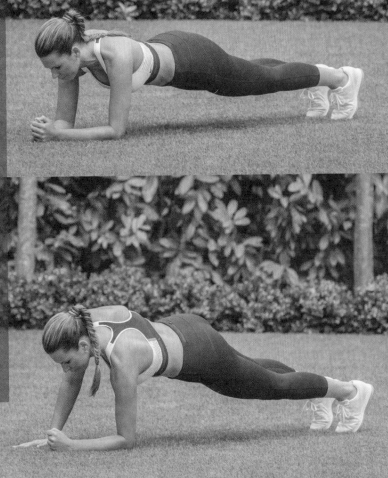

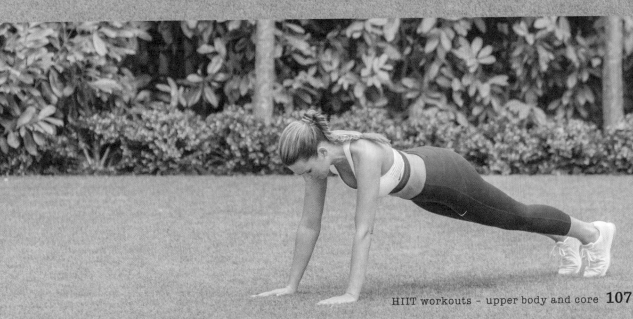

mountain climbers

WORK 30 SECONDS, **REST** 30 SECONDS

1 Start in a plank position with hands about shoulder-width apart, body straight, head aligned and core engaged.

2 Pull one knee into the chest, then switch to pull the other knee in. Repeat this movement.

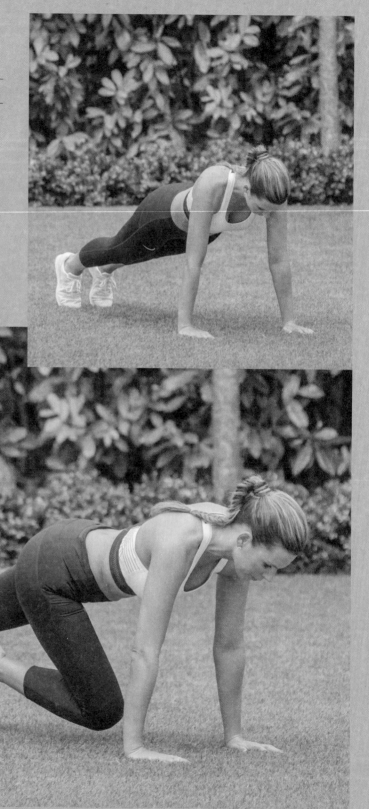

cross climbers

1 Start in a plank position with hands about shoulder-width apart, body straight, head aligned and core engaged.

2 Pull one knee into the chest and twist towards the opposite elbow. Alternate with the other leg.

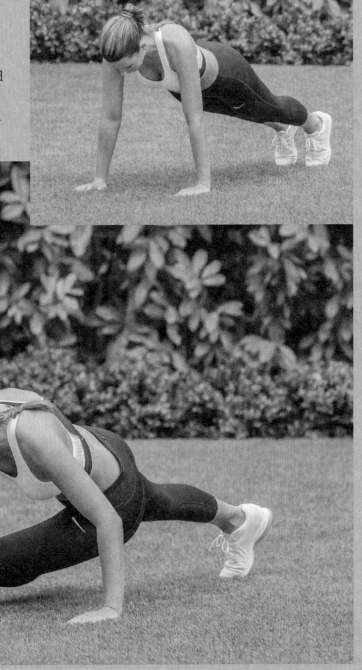

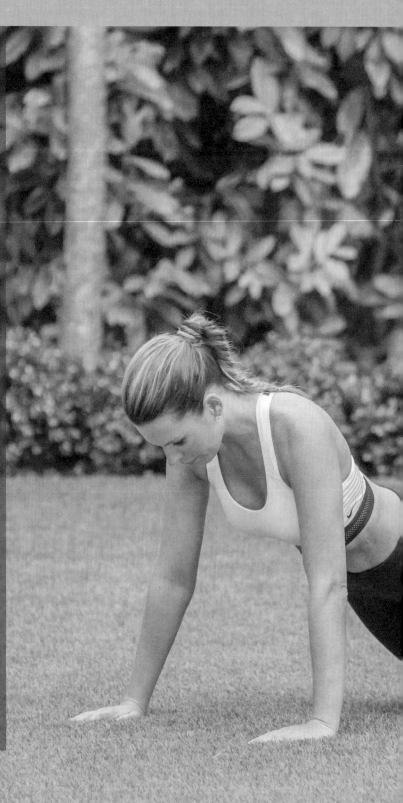

press-ups

WORK 30 SECONDS

REST 30 SECONDS

1 Begin in a press-up position with knees on the ground, lower legs crossed and feet raised, arms straight and hands a little wider than the shoulders.

2 Bend your elbows so your body lowers almost (but not fully) to the ground, then return to the starting position. Repeat, keeping your body straight and moving up and down in a controlled way.

ADVANCED Start in a press-up position, this time with legs straight and toes tucked under, arms straight and hands a little wider than the shoulders. Bend your elbows so your body lowers, then return to the starting position. Repeat, moving up and down in a controlled movement.

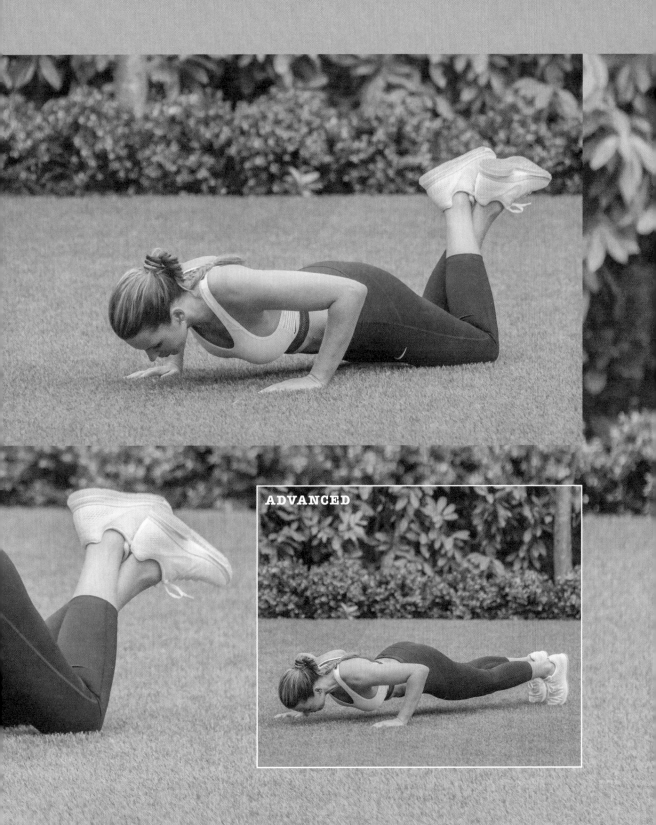

ADVANCED

burpees

WORK 30 SECONDS

REST 30 SECONDS

1 Start in a plank position, body straight, hands and feet about shoulder-width apart, toes tucked under.

2 Bring your knees into a crouching position.

3 Straighten your legs and jump upwards. Return to the crouching position and then back down to the plank position. Repeat.

ADVANCED Start face-down, with your body on the ground, elbows bent, hands under the shoulders. Bring your legs forwards and up into a crouching position, jump upwards and return to the starting position.

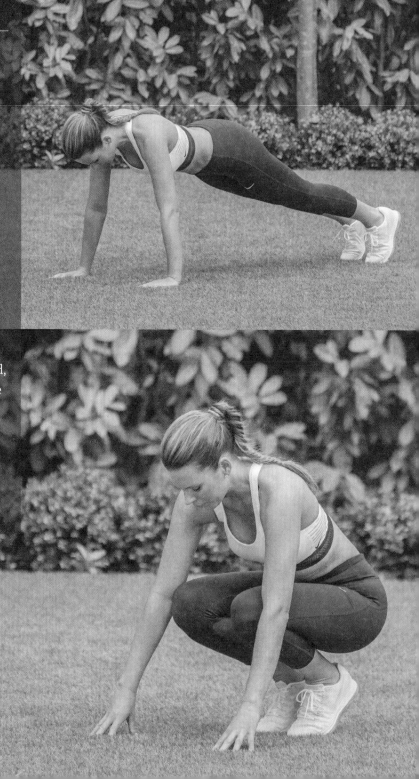

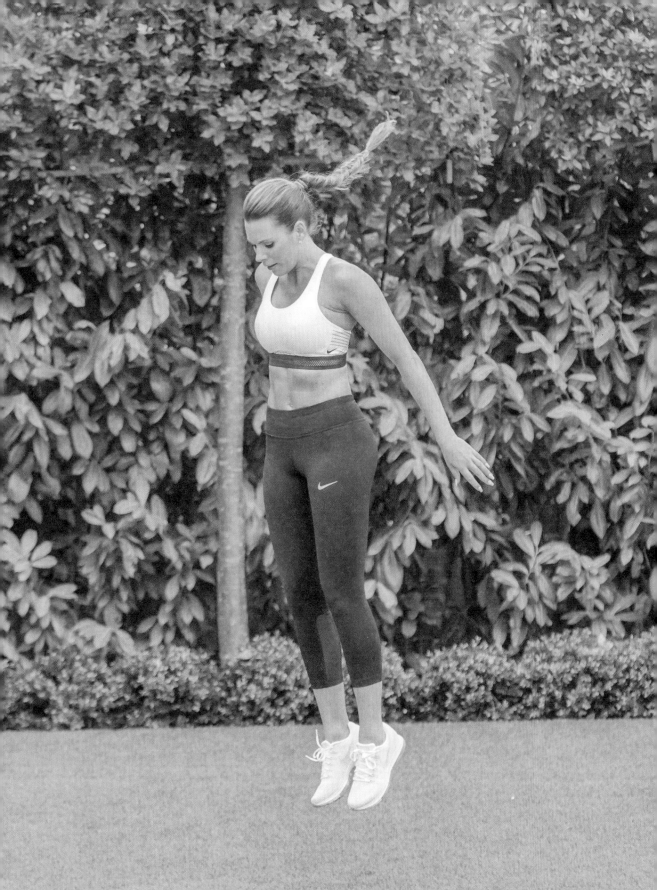

full body

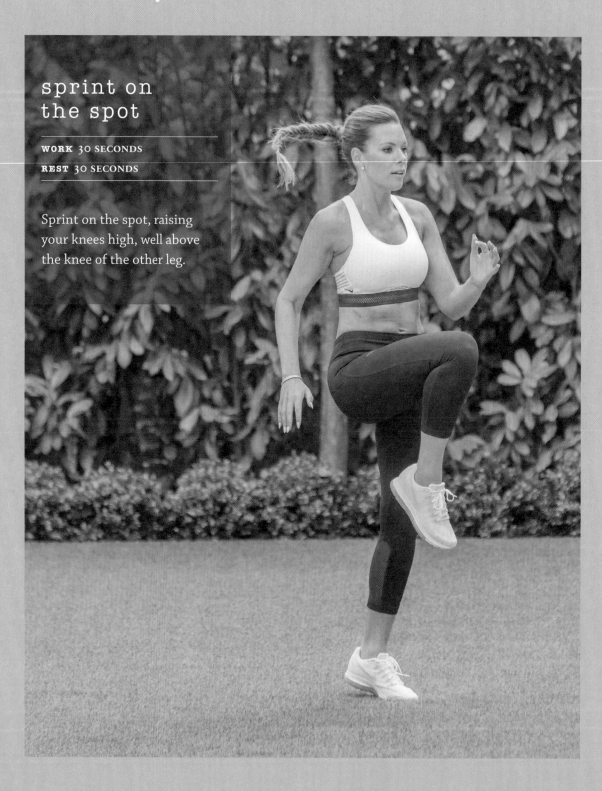

sprint on the spot

WORK 30 SECONDS

REST 30 SECONDS

Sprint on the spot, raising
your knees high, well above
the knee of the other leg.

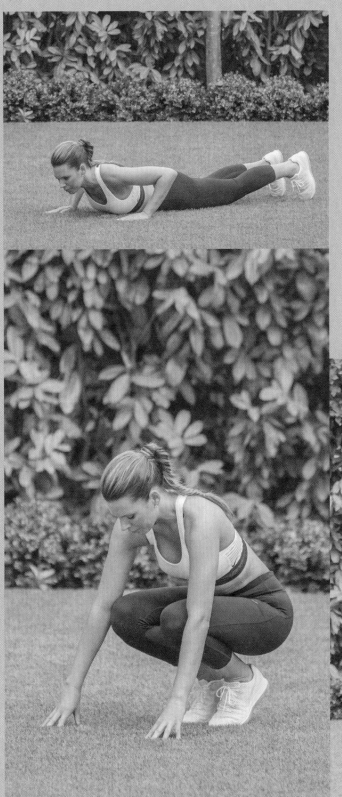

push-up burpees

WORK 30 SECONDS, **REST** 30 SECONDS

1 Start face down with your body on the ground, elbows bent, hands under the shoulders.

2 Bring your legs forwards and up into a crouching position.

3 Straighten your legs and jump upwards, then return to the crouching position, followed by the starting position. Repeat.

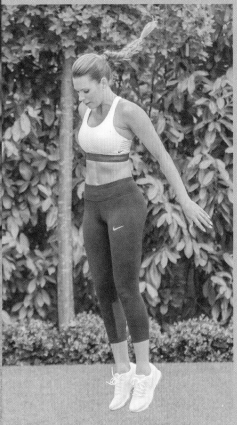

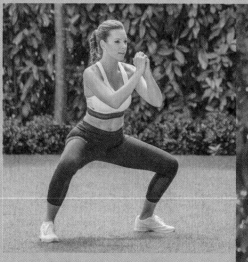

squat jumps

WORK 30 SECONDS, **REST** 30 SECONDS

1 From a standing position, squat down as if sitting on a chair behind you, keeping your core engaged and holding your hands in front for balance.

2 Throw your arms back and jump up. Come back down to the squat position and repeat.

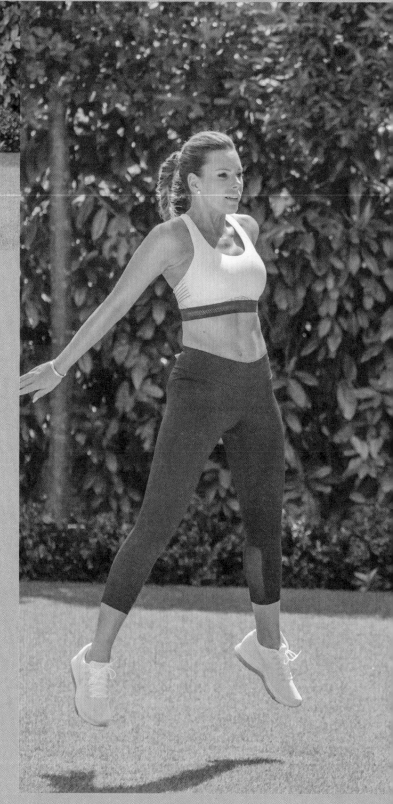

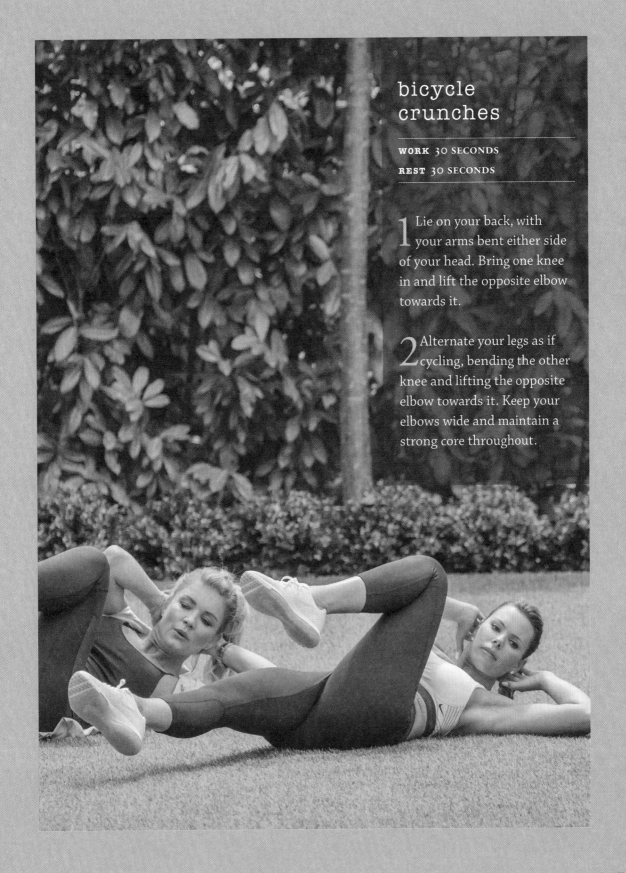

bicycle crunches

WORK 30 SECONDS
REST 30 SECONDS

1 Lie on your back, with your arms bent either side of your head. Bring one knee in and lift the opposite elbow towards it.

2 Alternate your legs as if cycling, bending the other knee and lifting the opposite elbow towards it. Keep your elbows wide and maintain a strong core throughout.

toe touch pikes

1 Start in a plank position.
Keeping your legs straight, push
back into an A position and touch
your left foot with your right hand.

2 Return to the plank position,
then repeat the same exercise,
this time touching your right foot
with your left hand.

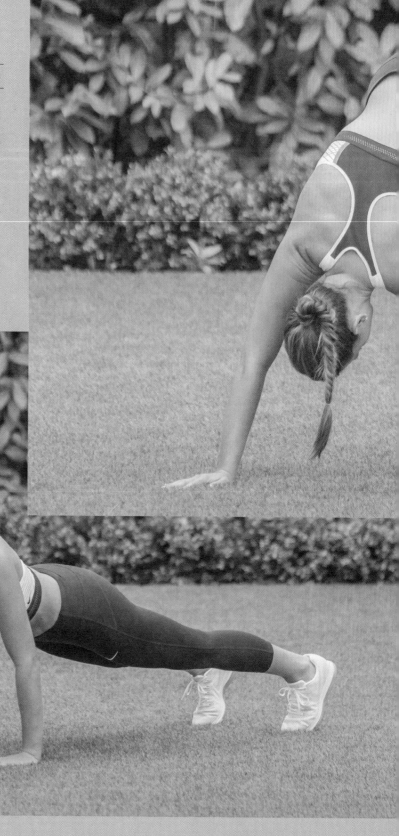

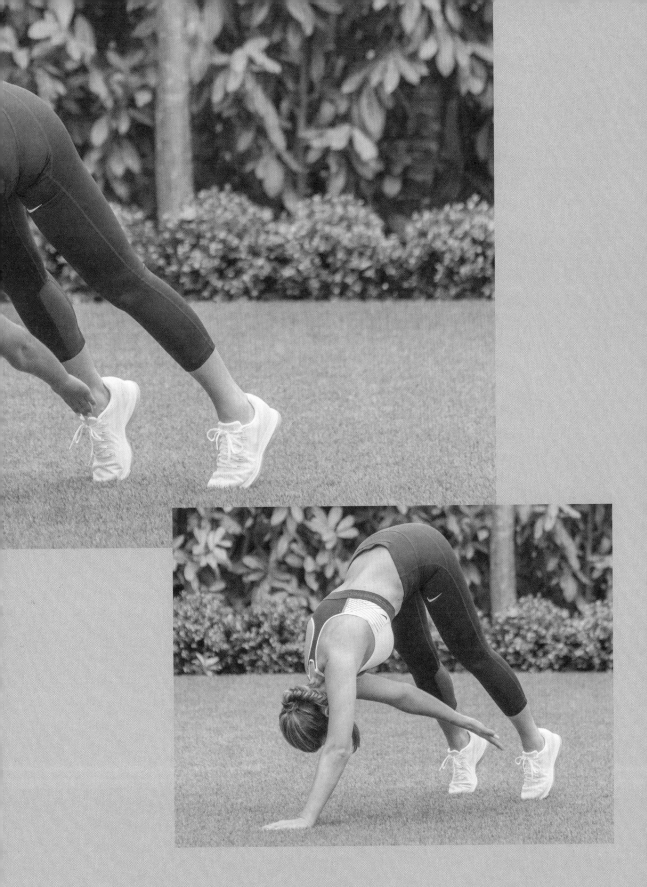

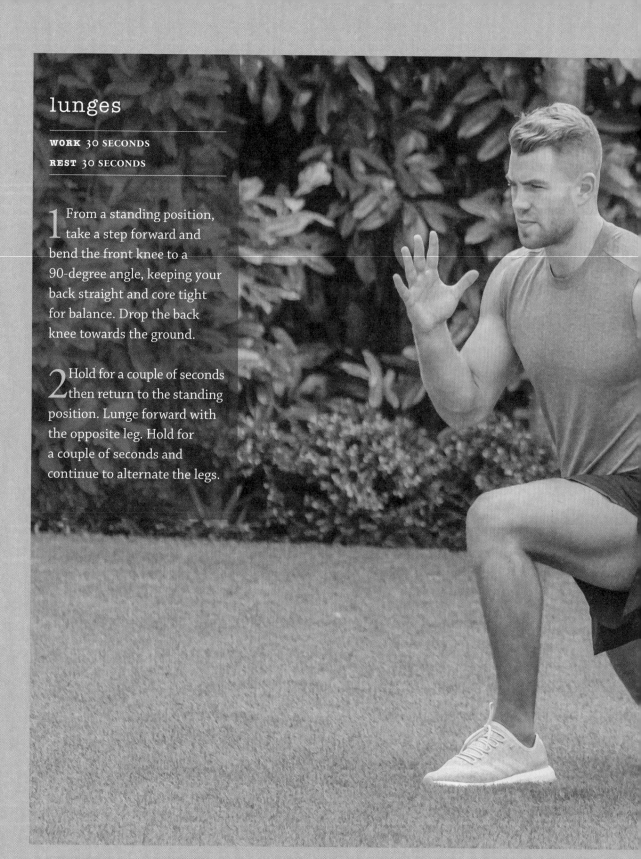

lunges

WORK 30 SECONDS

REST 30 SECONDS

1 From a standing position, take a step forward and bend the front knee to a 90-degree angle, keeping your back straight and core tight for balance. Drop the back knee towards the ground.

2 Hold for a couple of seconds then return to the standing position. Lunge forward with the opposite leg. Hold for a couple of seconds and continue to alternate the legs.

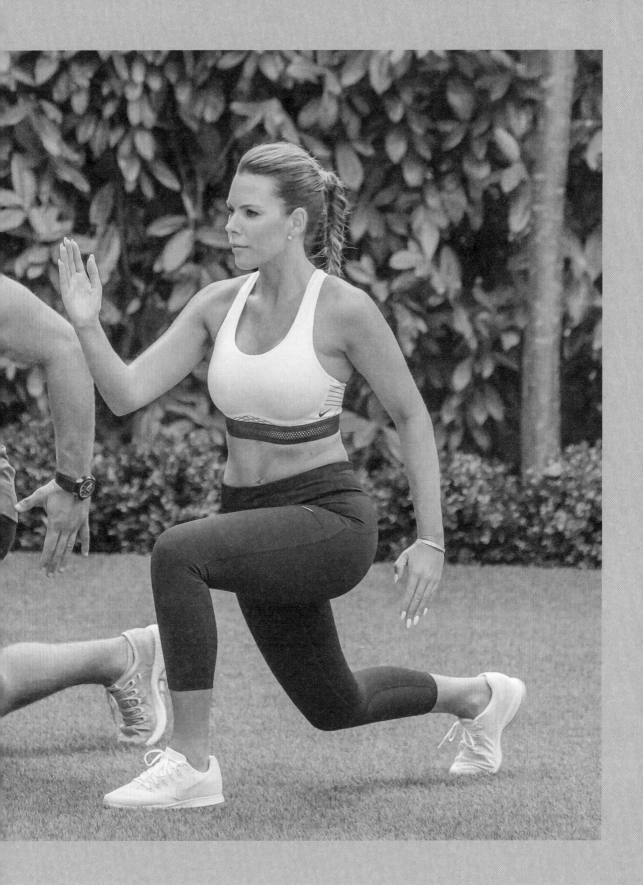

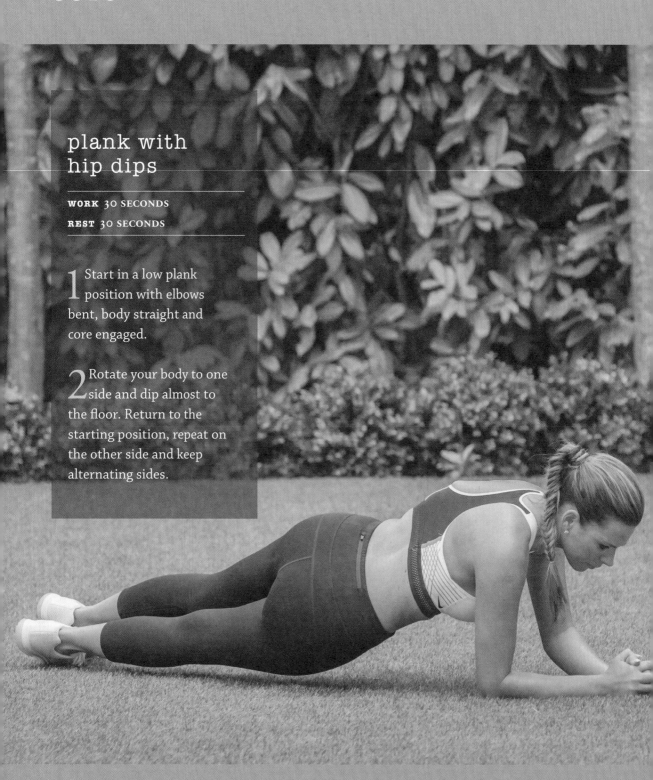

core

plank with
hip dips

WORK 30 SECONDS
REST 30 SECONDS

1 Start in a low plank position with elbows bent, body straight and core engaged.

2 Rotate your body to one side and dip almost to the floor. Return to the starting position, repeat on the other side and keep alternating sides.

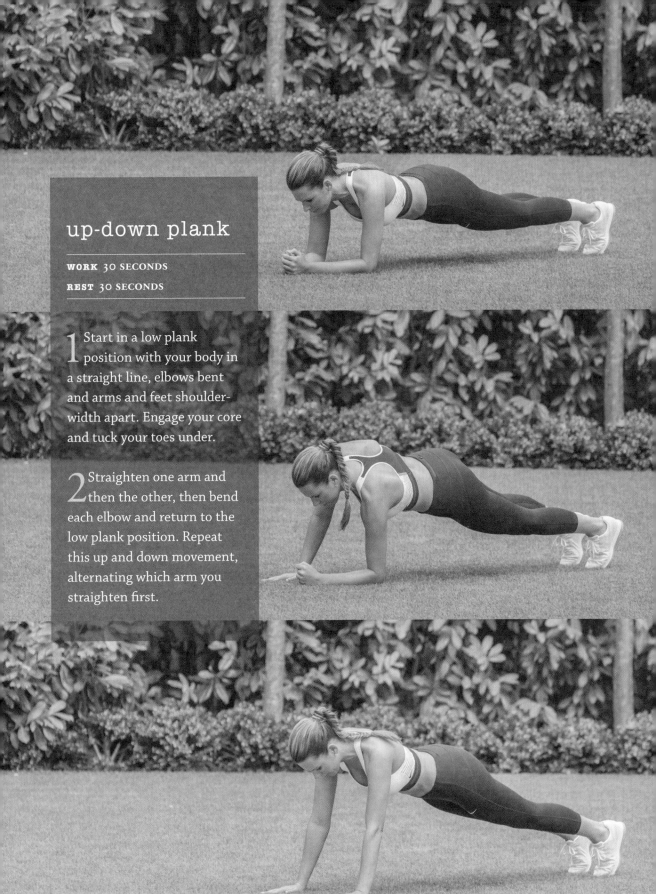

up-down plank

WORK 30 SECONDS

REST 30 SECONDS

1 Start in a low plank position with your body in a straight line, elbows bent and arms and feet shoulder-width apart. Engage your core and tuck your toes under.

2 Straighten one arm and then the other, then bend each elbow and return to the low plank position. Repeat this up and down movement, alternating which arm you straighten first.

cross climbers

WORK 30 SECONDS, **REST** 30 SECONDS

1 Start in a plank position with hands about shoulder-width apart, body straight, head aligned and core engaged.

2 Pull one knee into the chest and twist towards the opposite elbow. Alternate with the other leg.

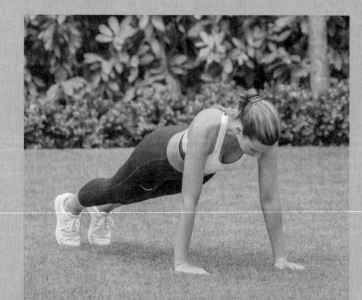

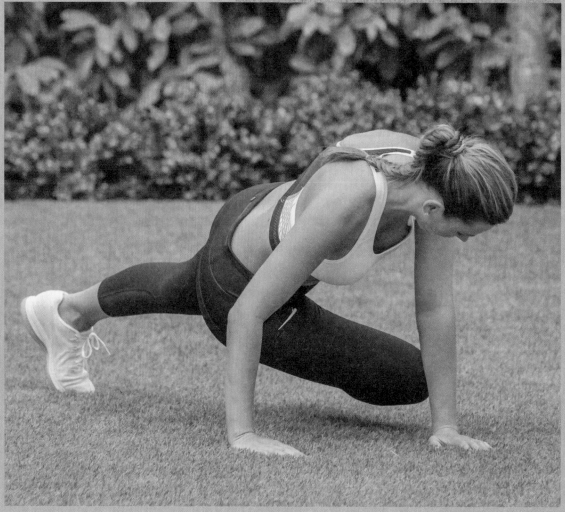

v-sit crunches

1 Begin sitting on the ground with legs bent, feet slightly raised and hands lightly touching the side of your head.

2 Stretch out your legs as you lower your upper body. Then return to the starting position, and repeat. Keep your elbows wide and maintain a strong core throughout.

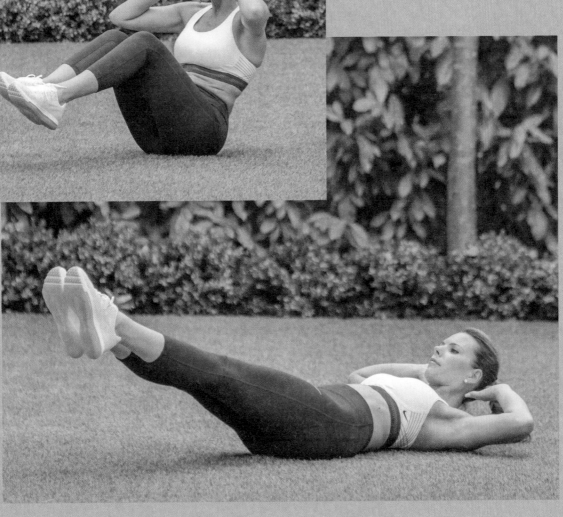

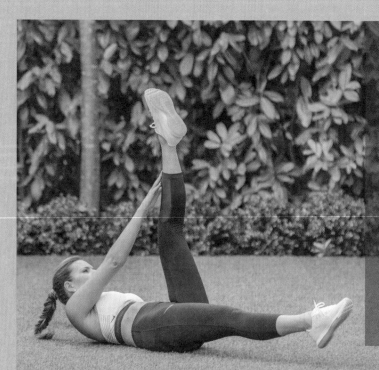

the toni

WORK 30 SECONDS
REST 30 SECONDS

Lie on the ground, raise one leg and reach for the foot with the opposite arm. Return to the starting position, then straighten the other leg and reach with the opposite arm. Repeat.

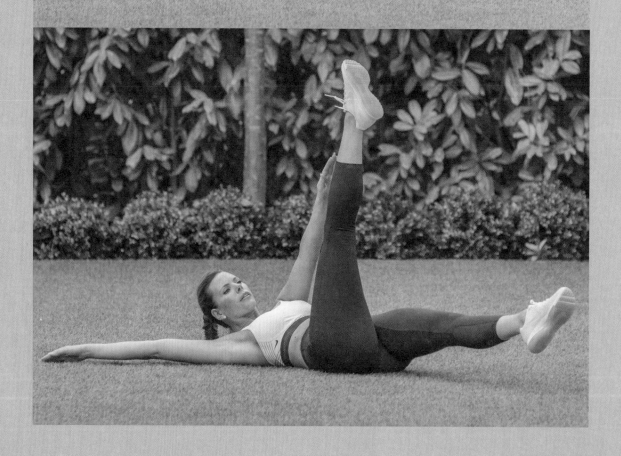

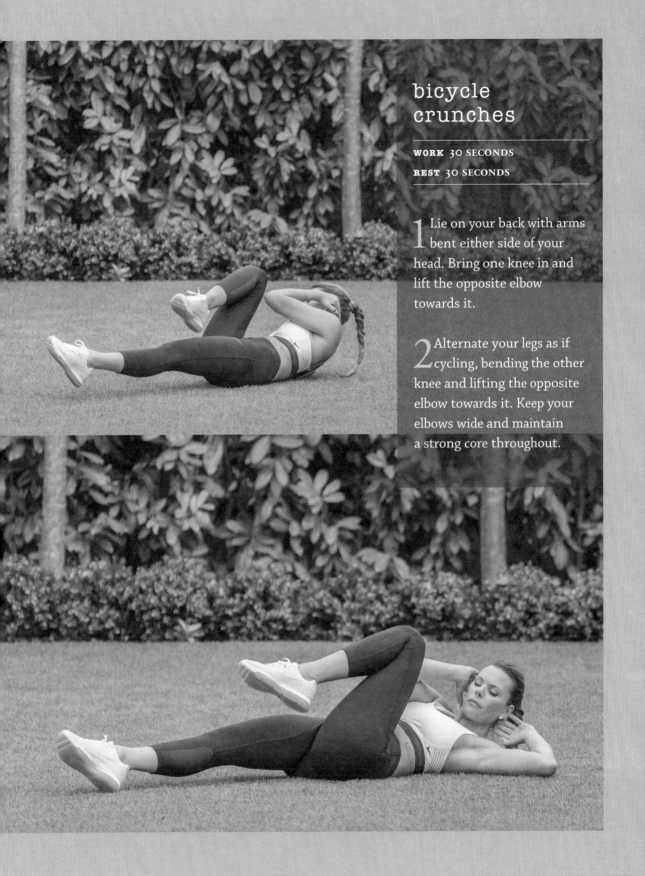

bicycle crunches

WORK 30 SECONDS

REST 30 SECONDS

1 Lie on your back with arms bent either side of your head. Bring one knee in and lift the opposite elbow towards it.

2 Alternate your legs as if cycling, bending the other knee and lifting the opposite elbow towards it. Keep your elbows wide and maintain a strong core throughout.

'burst' workouts

Alongside the more structured workouts I do every week, I also do quick 'burst' workouts, just a few minutes here and there when I'm brushing my teeth, cooking or just when I have some moments spare. (My family used to think I was slightly mad doing this but I think have got used to it now!) If you do a little bit every day then it does make a difference – so why not devise your own burst workouts? Here are a few ideas.

● Squats while you're cleaning your teeth – don't just stand there brushing your teeth, squat during those two minutes! Get nice white teeth AND a firm behind!

● Lunges while you're cooking or waiting for the kettle to boil. You could also do a few leg stretches while holding on to your kitchen work-top or table.

● Run up and down the stairs for five minutes, and do a few lunges on the bottom step to finish. (Careful, though, don't fall down the stairs!)

● Put on one song (preferably your favourite and one that gets you moving) and do a quick workout. This is a fun one to do with your buddies or family and will have you all giggling within moments. Try a few high-knee runs, squat jumps or stretches against some furniture, or just throw some moves. Before you know it your song will be over and you'll have done a 3-minute workout. If anything, you might have had a good laugh in the process!

● If you're standing in a queue or just waiting around to go out, you could tone those lower-leg muscles by doing a few calf raises. Put the balls of your feet on a step or a kerb and then raise your heels onto your tiptoes. Hold for a few seconds, then lower your heels.

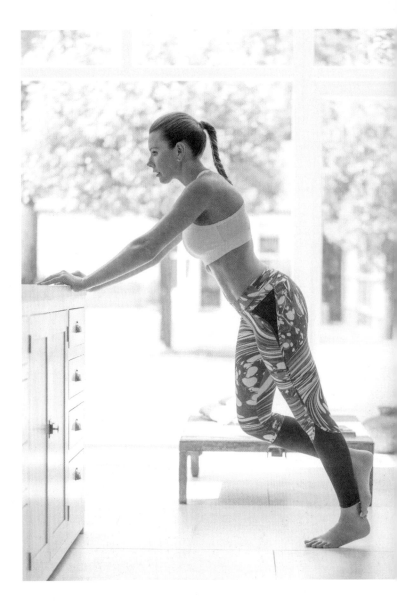

● Do a few stretches in the evening, in front of the TV or somewhere quiet. Try to slow down your breathing, calm your mind and really focus on what your body is doing. If you've done a tough workout that day why not congratulate yourself for getting through it. Learn to appreciate how amazing your body is and give it a bit of attention!

running

Cardio-based workouts are also a key part of my exercise routine. This kind of LISS (low-intensity steady state) training is performed over a longer period of time, it's less stressful on the body and improves your vascular fitness. Running makes a good cardio workout and I find it really calming for the mind. As I've got fitter I've increased the distance, speed and time that I run. Always warm up before a run with a brisk 5-minute walk.

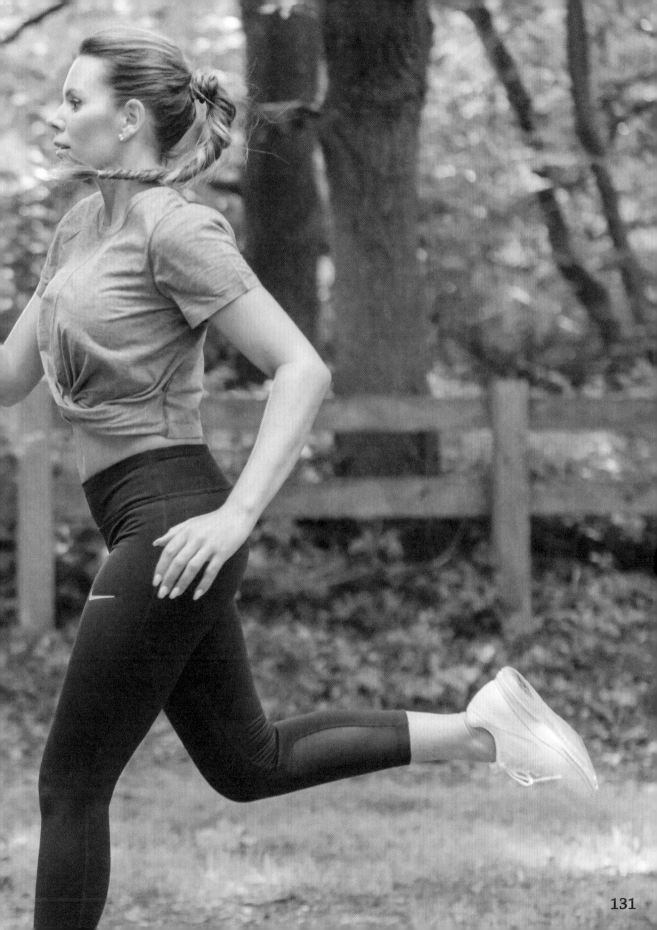

circuit training

Circuit training combines cardio and strength moves. It's a good fat-burning workout and helps you tone and gain lean muscle at the same time. You move quickly from one exercise to the other and it's great to do with your buddies. Do each exercise for 60 seconds followed by 60 seconds of rest, then move on to the next exercise. Complete five rounds and make sure your technique is correct throughout.

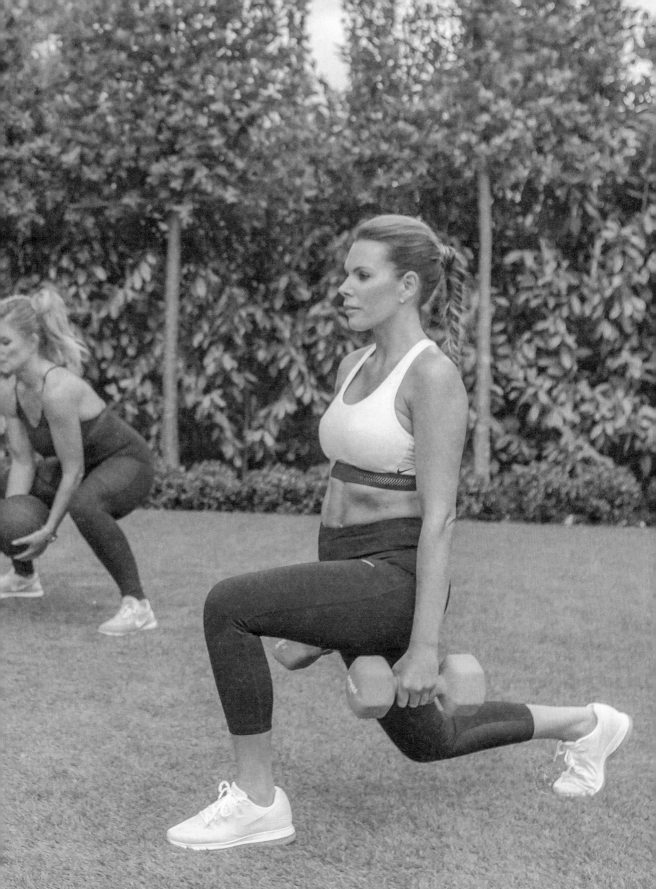

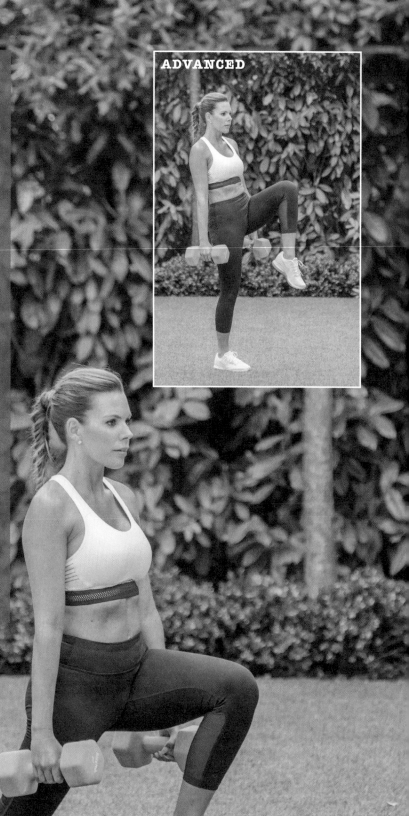

walking dumbbell lunges

WORK 60 SECONDS
REST 60 SECONDS

1 Stand in an upright position holding a dumbbell in each hand. Step forward into a lunge position with your knees at an approximate 90-degree angle. Return to a standing position and repeat with the opposite leg. Keep the movement flowing.

ADVANCED As you step forward from standing, raise one knee, driving it from your glutes and then step forward with the same knee. Return to the standing position and repeat with the opposite leg.

ADVANCED

slam ball slams

WORK 60 SECONDS

REST 60 SECONDS

1 With your knees slightly wider than your shoulders, bend down and pick up the slam ball, keeping your back straight.

2 Bring the ball up to chest height with your knees still bent and back straight.

3 Return to an upright position with the ball at chest height.

4 Raise the ball above your head.

5 Bend the knees and slam the ball down in front of you with aggression. Repeat.

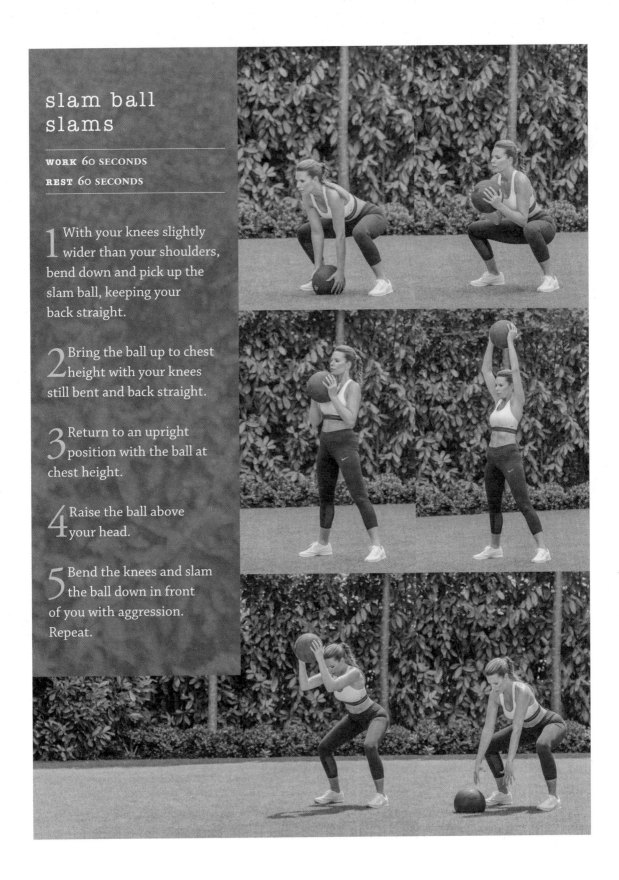

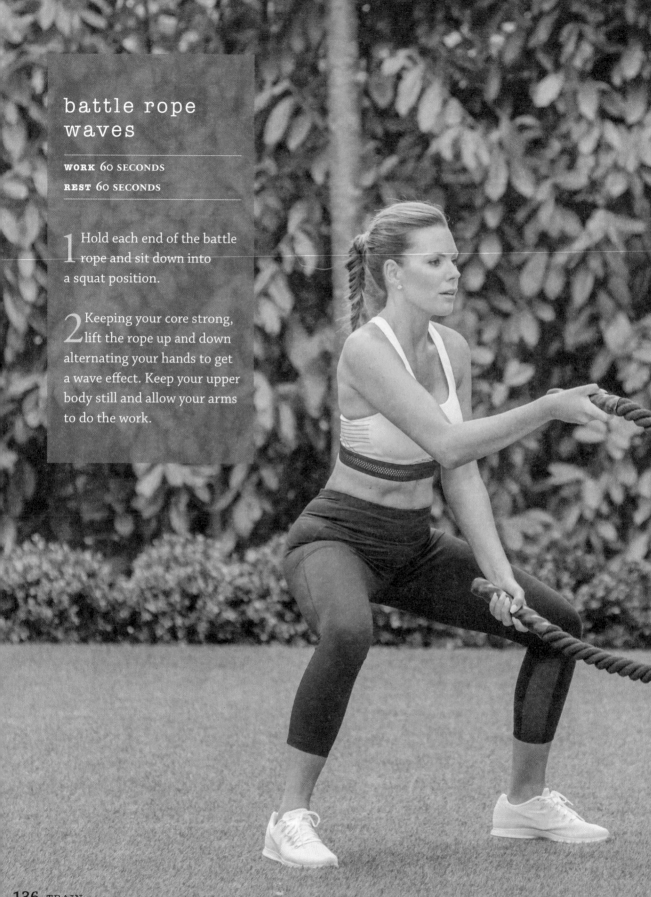

battle rope waves

WORK 60 SECONDS
REST 60 SECONDS

1 Hold each end of the battle rope and sit down into a squat position.

2 Keeping your core strong, lift the rope up and down alternating your hands to get a wave effect. Keep your upper body still and allow your arms to do the work.

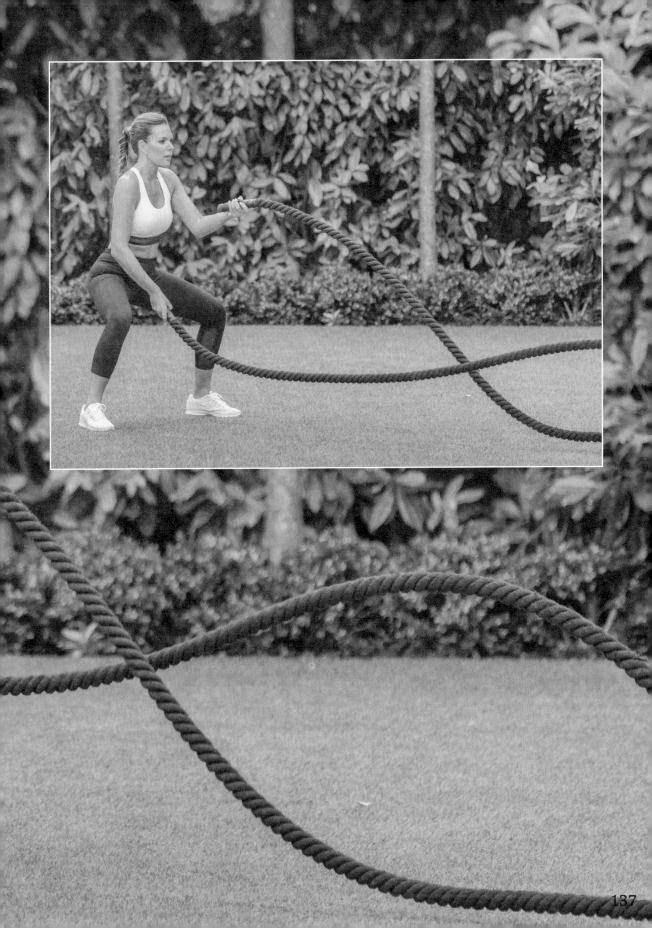

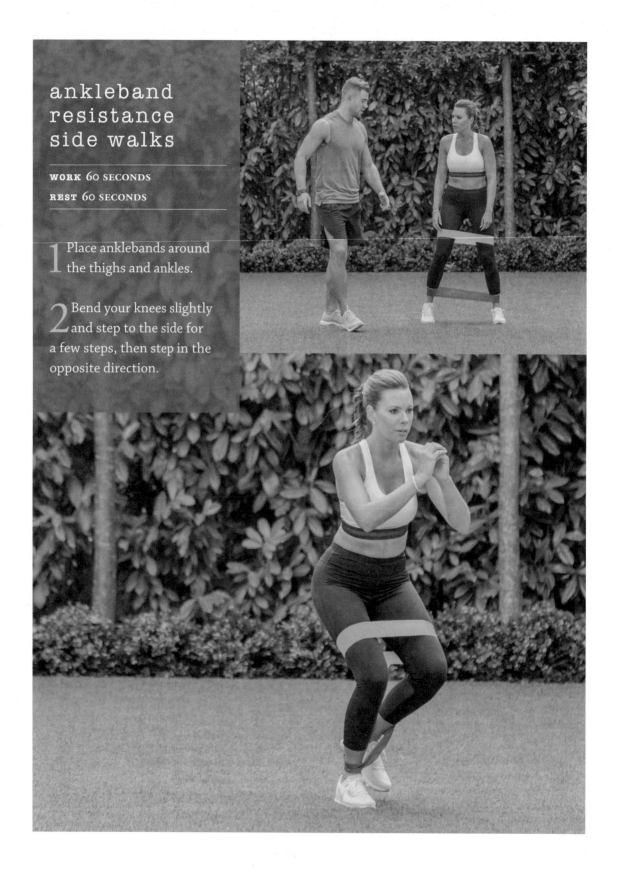

ankleband resistance side walks

WORK 60 SECONDS
REST 60 SECONDS

1 Place anklebands around the thighs and ankles.

2 Bend your knees slightly and step to the side for a few steps, then step in the opposite direction.

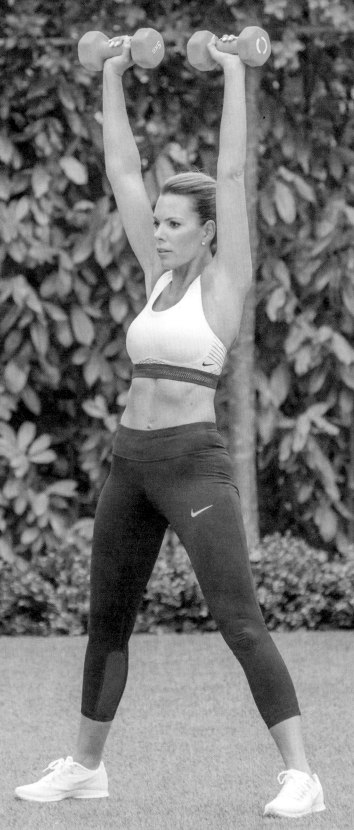

dumbbell squat and press

WORK 60 SECONDS
REST 60 SECONDS

1 Start in a squat position, knees bent, feet wider than shoulder-width and back straight. Balance the weights on your shoulders.

2 Drive from your heels, using your glutes to lift the weights into a shoulder raise. Return to the squat position and repeat.

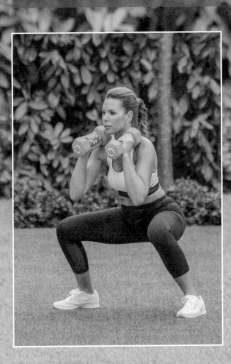

family activities

Of course, my best buddies are John and the children and we're often out and about playing games, walking the dogs and having fun. These everyday activities are as important as any exercise programme; the kids love it and we're all keeping active and healthy.

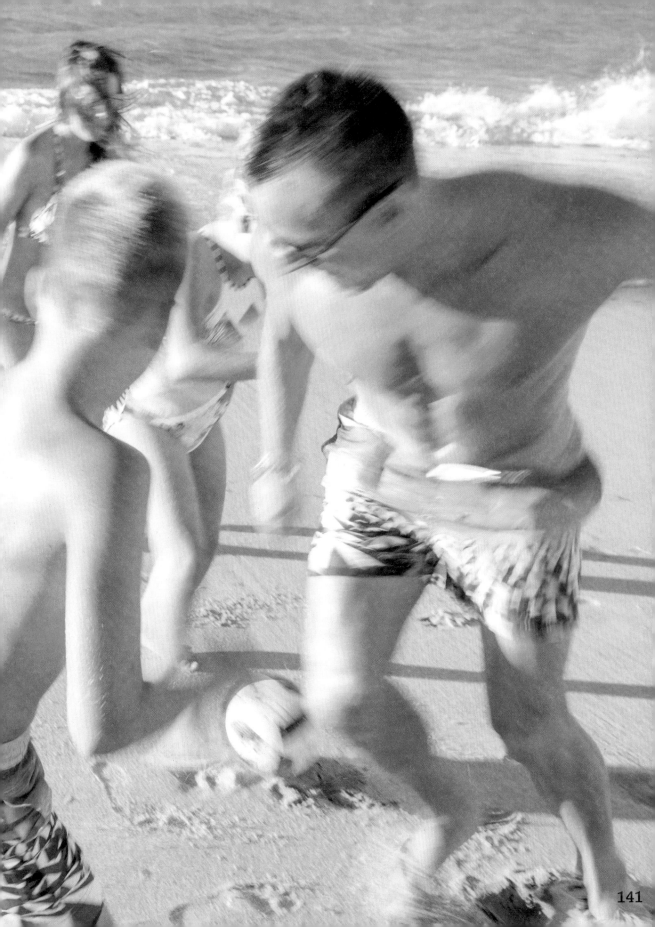

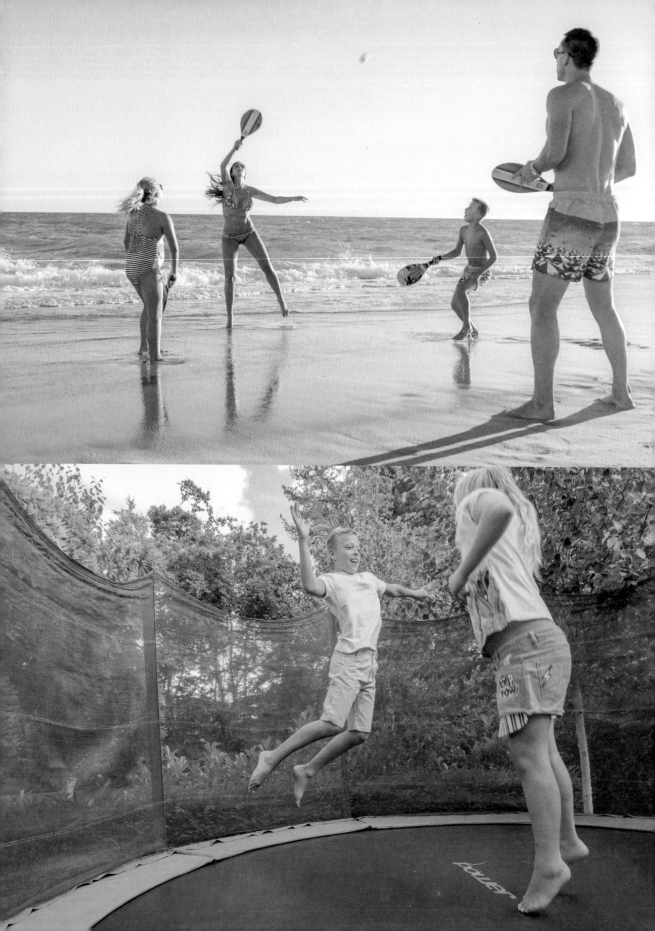

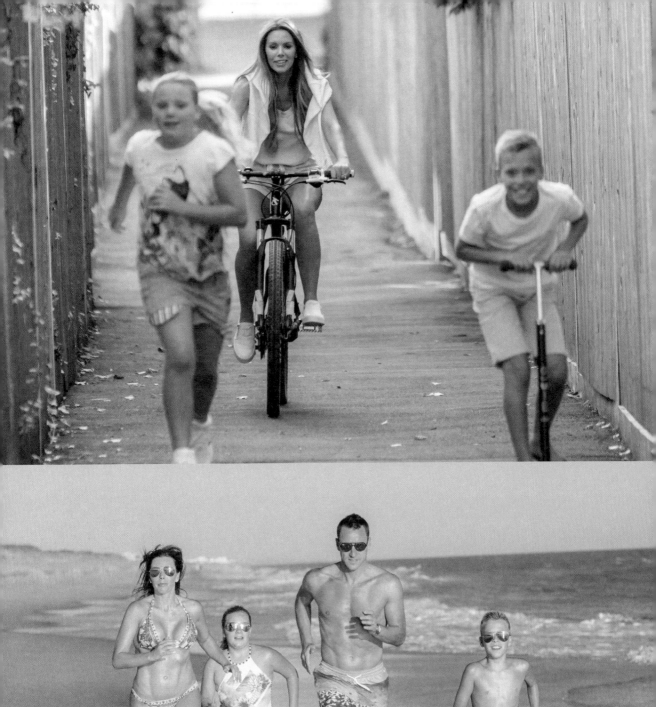
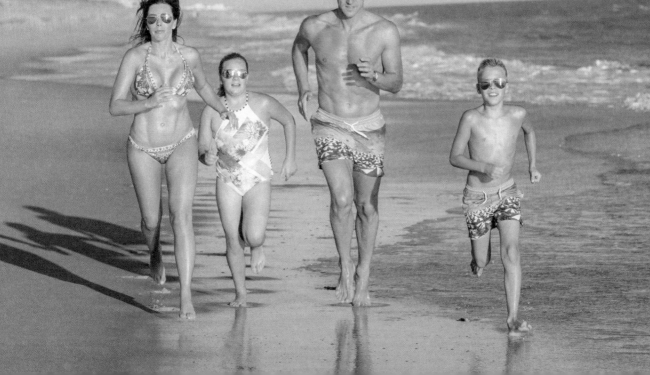

stretching

After every workout you need to cool down and stretch. Stretching helps to relax your muscles, improves flexibility, reduces the risk of injury and calms the mind. I recommend stretching for 5–10 minutes after a workout.

Target the areas of the body you've been working, hold each stretch for 30 seconds and repeat the stretch twice. Really focus on the stretch you're doing and slow your breathing.

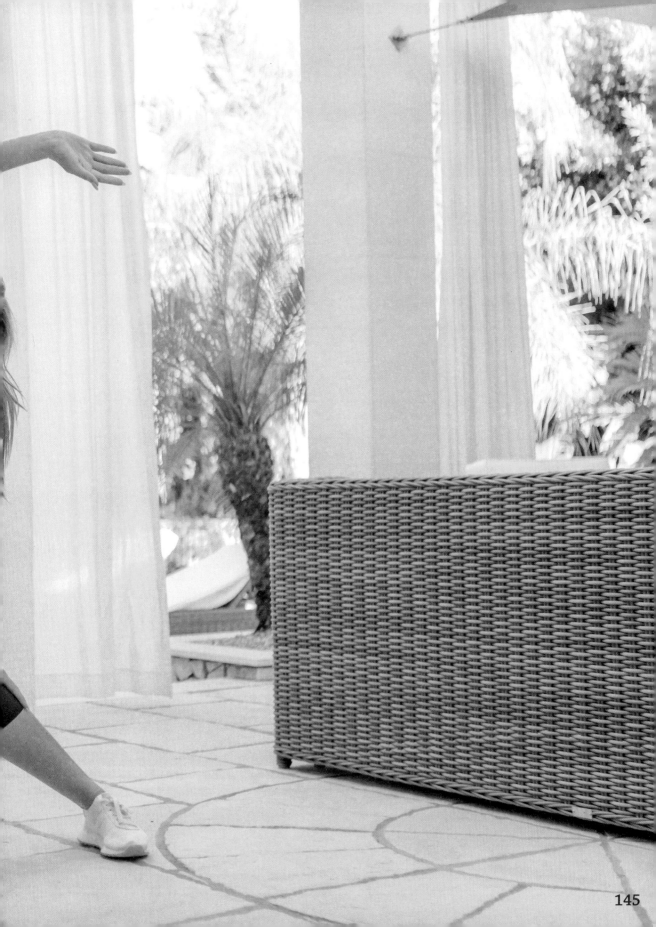

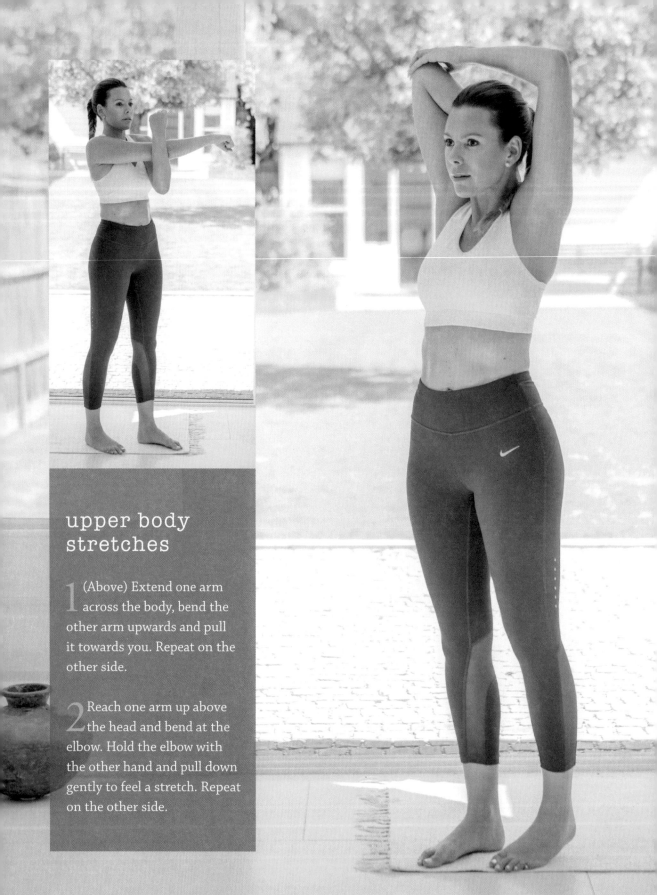

upper body stretches

1 (Above) Extend one arm across the body, bend the other arm upwards and pull it towards you. Repeat on the other side.

2 Reach one arm up above the head and bend at the elbow. Hold the elbow with the other hand and pull down gently to feel a stretch. Repeat on the other side.

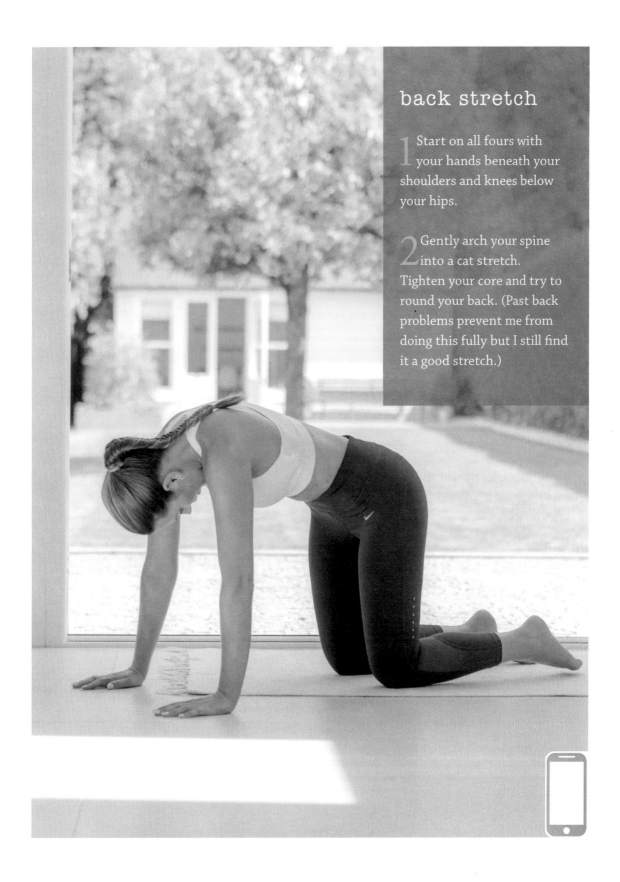

back stretch

1 Start on all fours with your hands beneath your shoulders and knees below your hips.

2 Gently arch your spine into a cat stretch. Tighten your core and try to round your back. (Past back problems prevent me from doing this fully but I still find it a good stretch.)

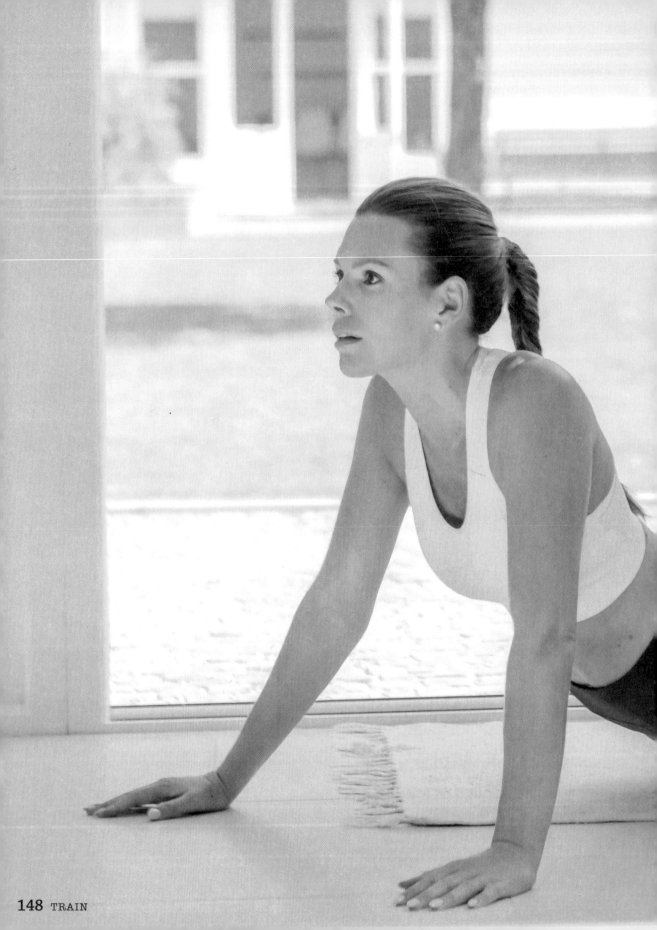

lower back stretches

1 Lie on your stomach with your legs extended and arms bent, your elbows under your shoulders and palms flat on the floor.

2 Gently push up into a cobra stretch by straightening your arms and lifting your upper body off the ground until you feel a good stretch in your lower back.

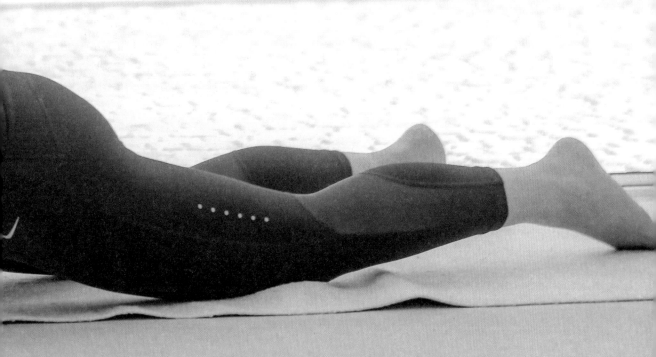

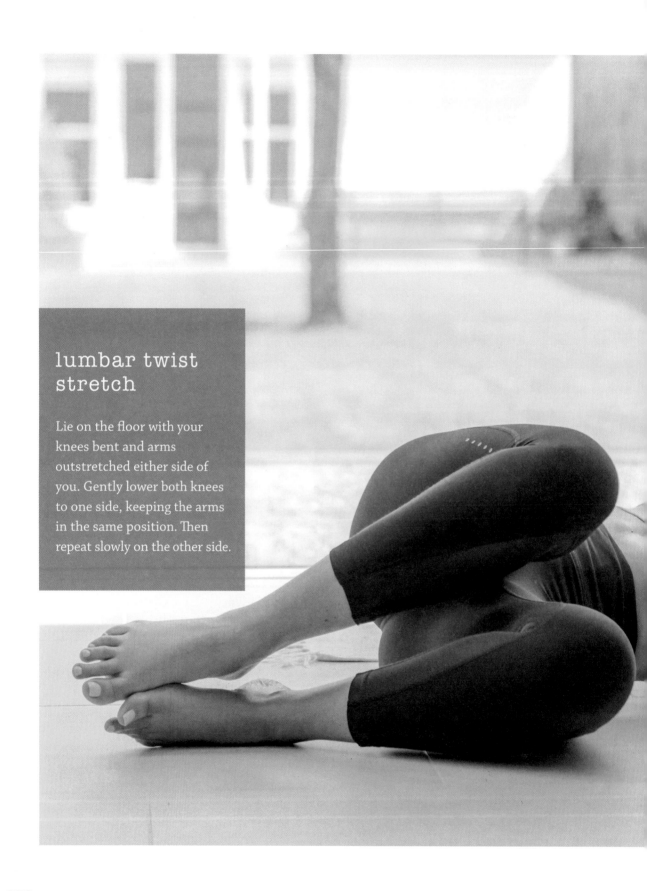

lumbar twist stretch

Lie on the floor with your knees bent and arms outstretched either side of you. Gently lower both knees to one side, keeping the arms in the same position. Then repeat slowly on the other side.

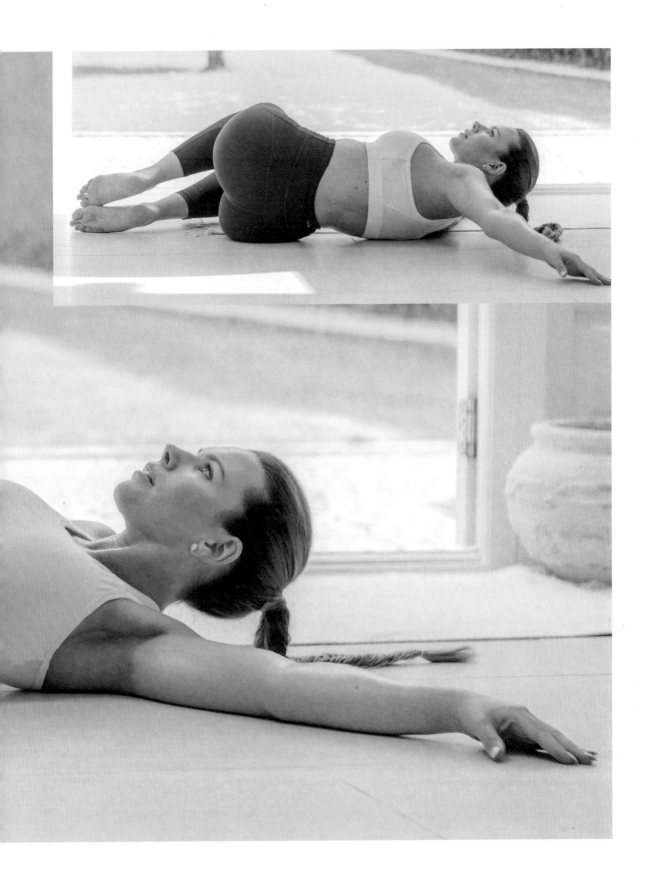

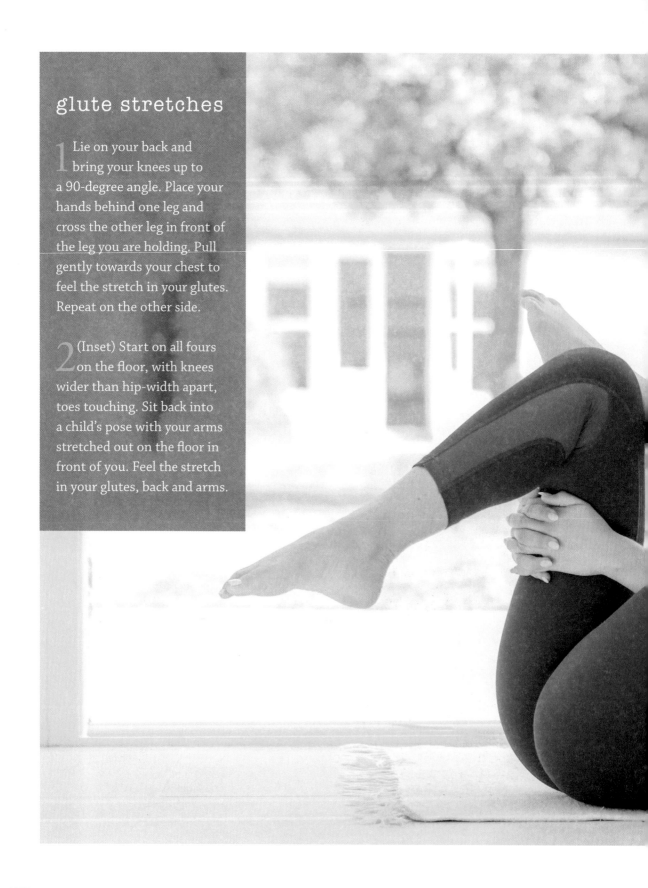

glute stretches

1 Lie on your back and bring your knees up to a 90-degree angle. Place your hands behind one leg and cross the other leg in front of the leg you are holding. Pull gently towards your chest to feel the stretch in your glutes. Repeat on the other side.

2 (Inset) Start on all fours on the floor, with knees wider than hip-width apart, toes touching. Sit back into a child's pose with your arms stretched out on the floor in front of you. Feel the stretch in your glutes, back and arms.

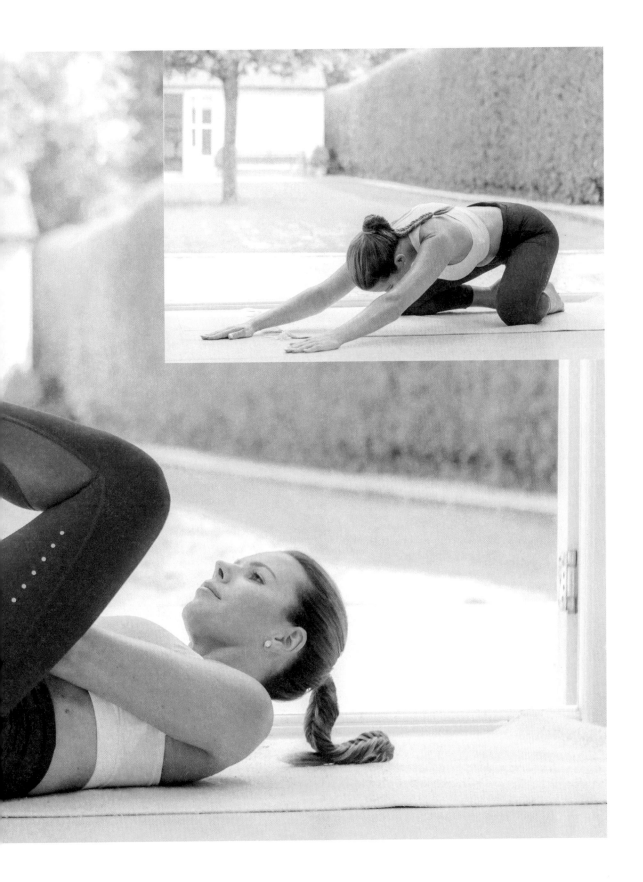

stretching **153**

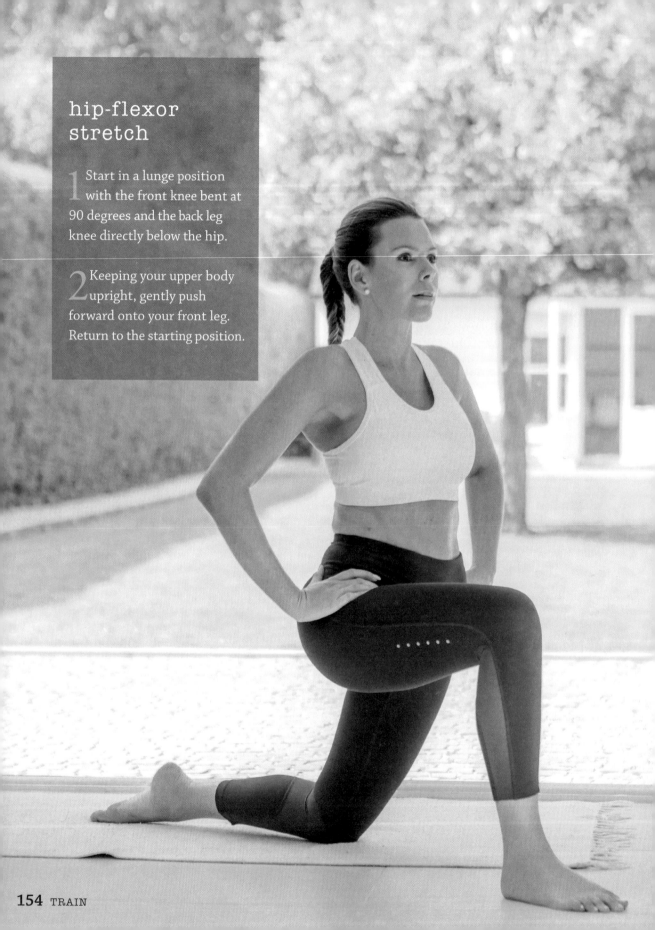

hip-flexor stretch

1 Start in a lunge position with the front knee bent at 90 degrees and the back leg knee directly below the hip.

2 Keeping your upper body upright, gently push forward onto your front leg. Return to the starting position.

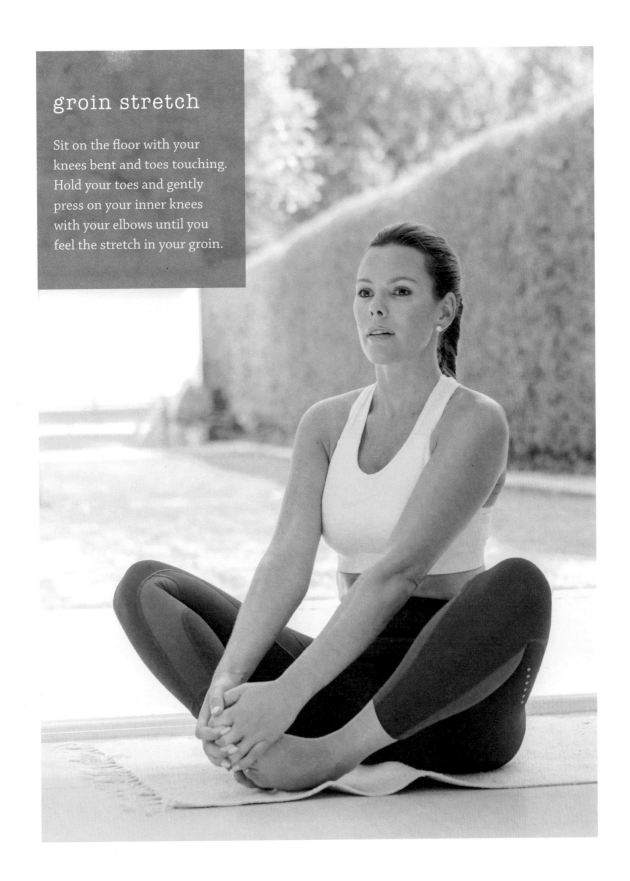

groin stretch

Sit on the floor with your knees bent and toes touching. Hold your toes and gently press on your inner knees with your elbows until you feel the stretch in your groin.

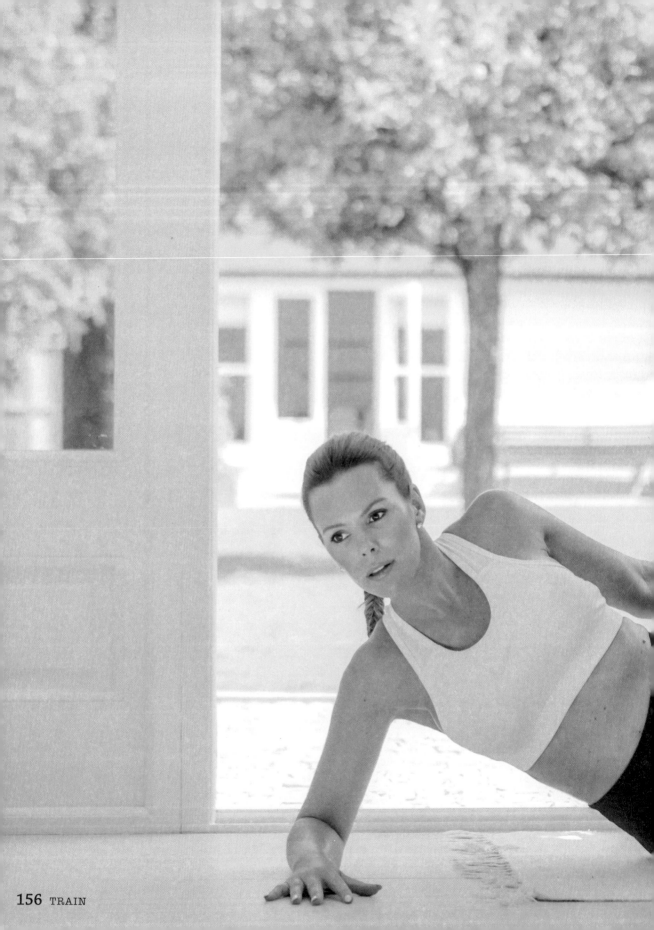

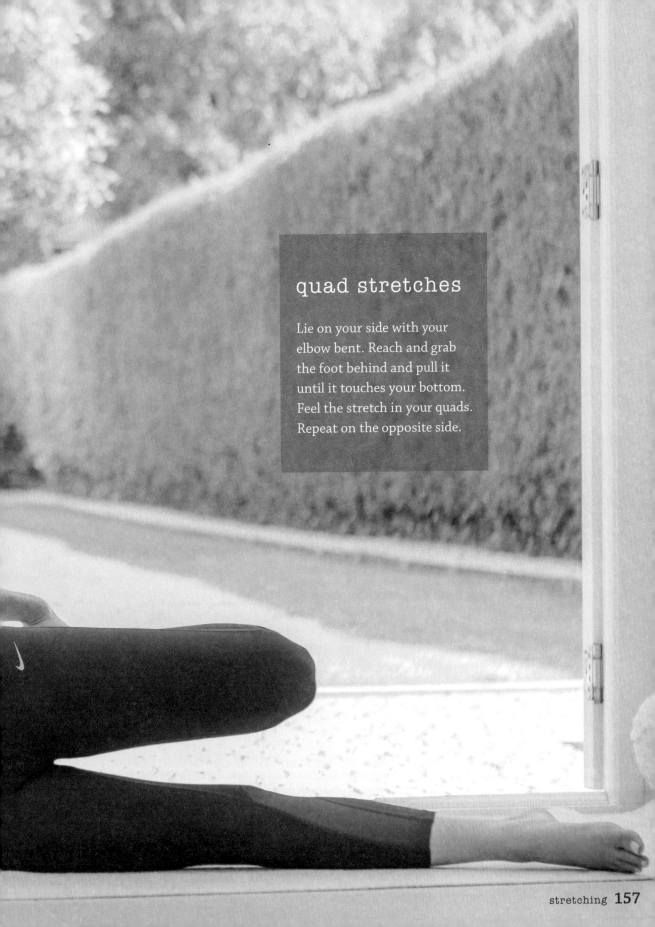

quad stretches

Lie on your side with your
elbow bent. Reach and grab
the foot behind and pull it
until it touches your bottom.
Feel the stretch in your quads.
Repeat on the opposite side.

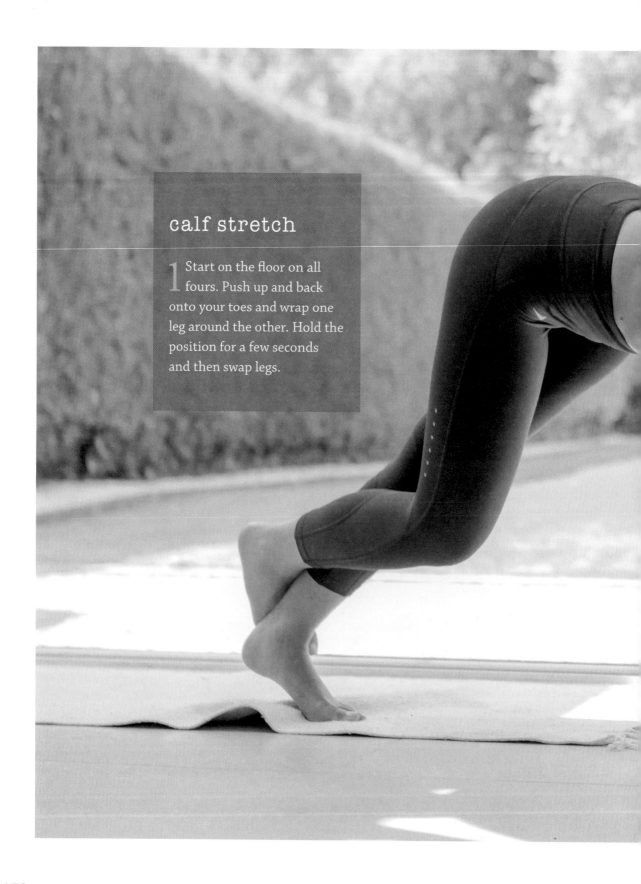

calf stretch

1 Start on the floor on all fours. Push up and back onto your toes and wrap one leg around the other. Hold the position for a few seconds and then swap legs.

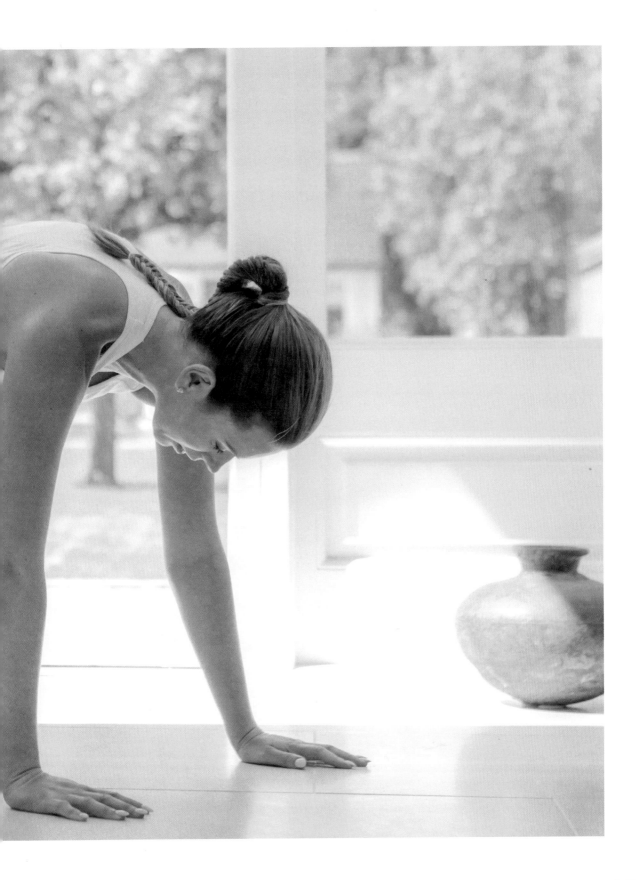

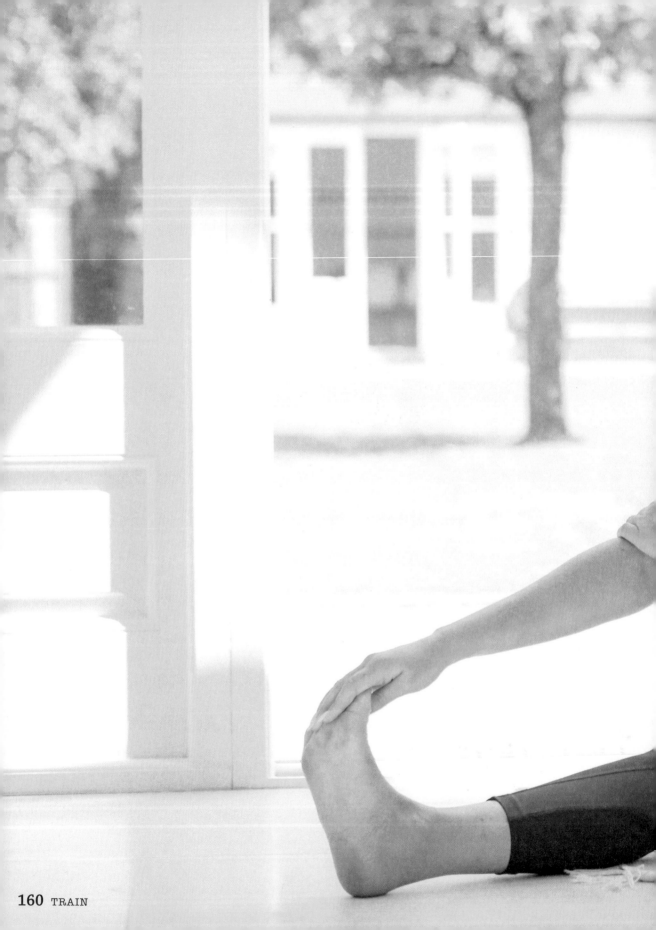

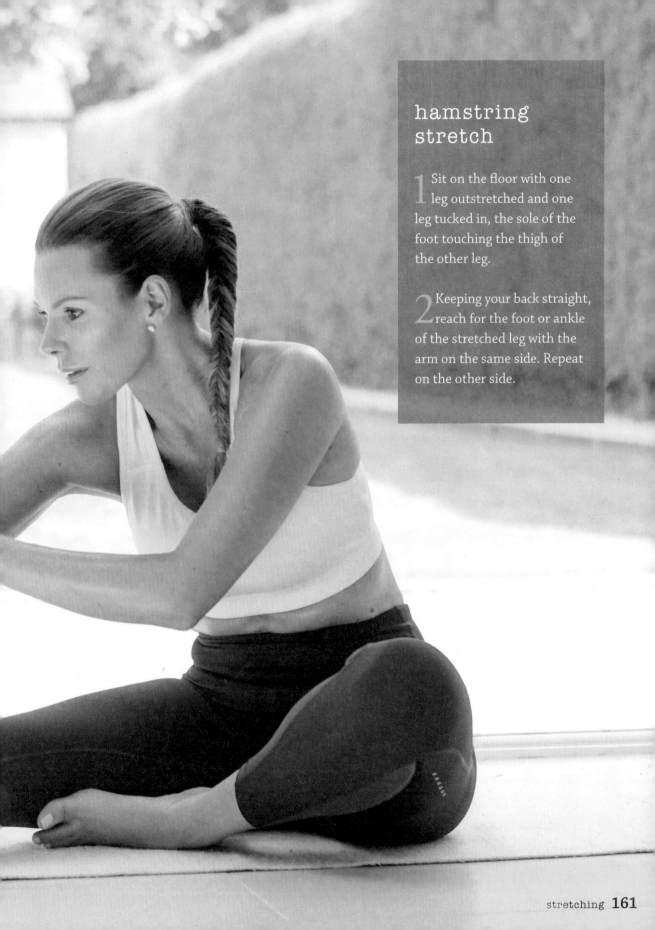

hamstring stretch

1 Sit on the floor with one leg outstretched and one leg tucked in, the sole of the foot touching the thigh of the other leg.

2 Keeping your back straight, reach for the foot or ankle of the stretched leg with the arm on the same side. Repeat on the other side.

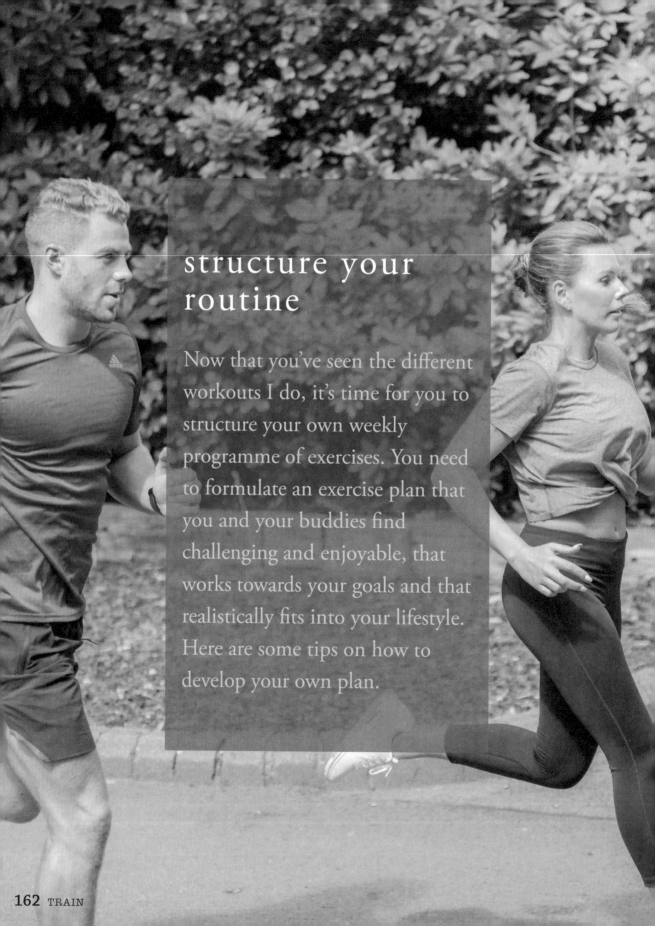

structure your routine

Now that you've seen the different workouts I do, it's time for you to structure your own weekly programme of exercises. You need to formulate an exercise plan that you and your buddies find challenging and enjoyable, that works towards your goals and that realistically fits into your lifestyle. Here are some tips on how to develop your own plan.

TRAINING SESSIONS PER WEEK

If you're a complete beginner, you might want to start with two to three workouts a week and build from there. Those new to exercise can sometimes set out with grand plans to work out every day, which can prove unachievable and unhealthy in the long term. Trainers often recommend four sessions a week and I currently do five a week, made up of HIIT and partner workouts, circuits and running (see my schedule overleaf). You need to think realistically about the number of days you can commit to training, but also develop a programme that pushes you sufficiently to achieve your goals. If you're working out with buddies, figure out when exactly you can meet up to train every week and stick to it – no excuses!

TYPES OF TRAINING

It's up to you to decide which types of exercise you want to do, depending on what works for you and your buddies and helps you to achieve your goals. I love HIIT workouts as they're intense and quick sessions that really boost cardiovascular fitness and work the body hard. As you move from one exercise to the other quickly, time seems to zip by. Partner workouts are fun and you can really motivate each other to get through each session. Circuits are great for fat-burning and toning muscle, whereas cardio LISS training improves general fitness levels and results in a leaner look. I do a combination of workouts and will sometimes vary things week to week just to ensure I never lose motivation.

PROGRESSION

Your aim with each session is to push yourself as that's the only way you'll improve, progress and see changes in your body. Each session should be a challenge; not so much that you injure yourself, but enough that you're pushing yourself hard and increasingly working above and beyond what you've previously done. As soon as an exercise feels comfortable or easier, then it's probably time to work harder. You can do this in a variety of ways: work out for longer and reduce the rest times in between, do more sets and rounds of exercises, try more advanced versions of some exercises, increase the number of sessions you do a week or vary the types of exercises you do.

I also advise keeping notes on your workouts, such as how many reps, sets or rounds you've managed or the distance and time you've achieved in a cardio workout, etc. Not only will keeping a record help you to see how you've improved but it will also motivate you to work harder.

BUMPS ALONG THE WAY

Sometimes, life gets in the way and you're forced to miss a training session or two. It happens to all of us and there's no need to panic or – heaven forbid – give up. Simply get back into your routine as soon as you can. If you're forced to miss a session, you might be able to fit in a few 'burst workouts' (see page 128), do a few stretches or go for a quick walk. And do keep eating healthily on any days off. If you've had to stop for a while, you might not be able to pick up from exactly where you left off but the sooner you return to your exercise routine, the sooner you'll be back on track.

WHEN WILL YOU SEE RESULTS?

This is the million-dollar question. Your body is not going to change overnight and you need to view exercising and eating well as more of a long-term lifestyle change, one that you integrate into your everyday life. If you eat well and stick to your exercise plan, pushing yourself hard, you should notice a change in your body shape after 12 weeks. Saying that, some people find that after four weeks of hard work their friends start to notice a difference, after eight weeks their family can see a change, and then after 12 weeks you (often the harshest critic) can see definite results in your body shape.

Here's an example of a typical week in my training schedule, just to give you an idea of how you might formulate your own weekly schedule now or in the future. I vary my workouts from week to week, and might replace one session with running or a partner workout, etc. I also do a good warm-up and cool down before and after each workout.

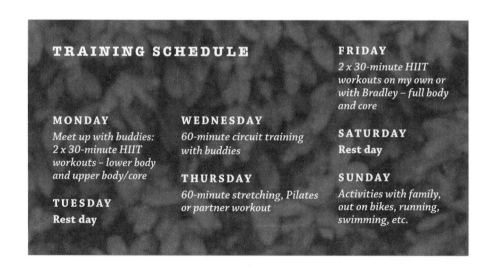

TRAINING SCHEDULE

MONDAY
Meet up with buddies: 2 x 30-minute HIIT workouts – lower body and upper body/core

TUESDAY
Rest day

WEDNESDAY
60-minute circuit training with buddies

THURSDAY
60-minute stretching, Pilates or partner workout

FRIDAY
2 x 30-minute HIIT workouts on my own or with Bradley – full body and core

SATURDAY
Rest day

SUNDAY
Activities with family, out on bikes, running, swimming, etc.

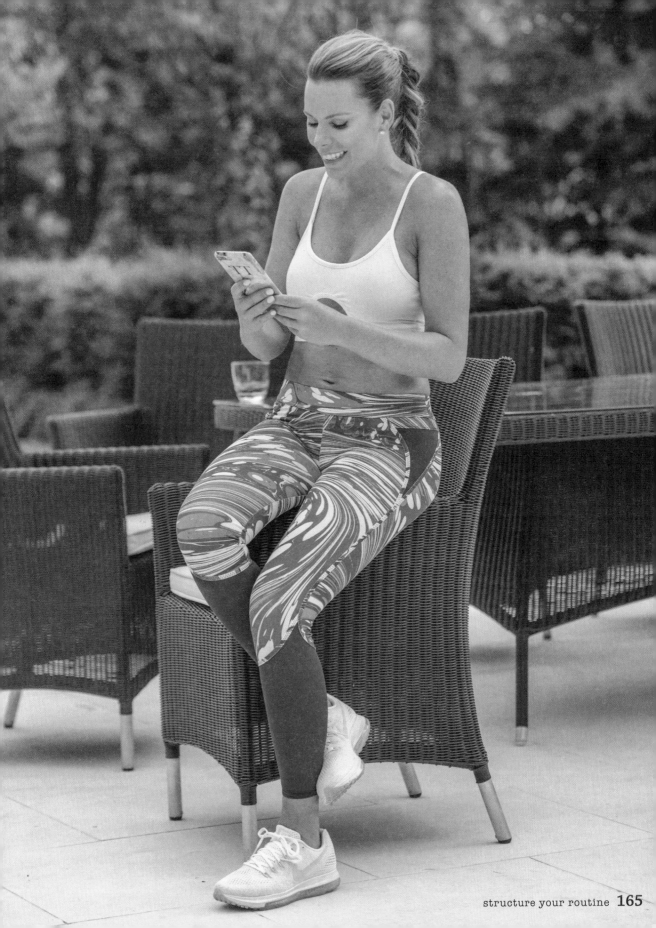

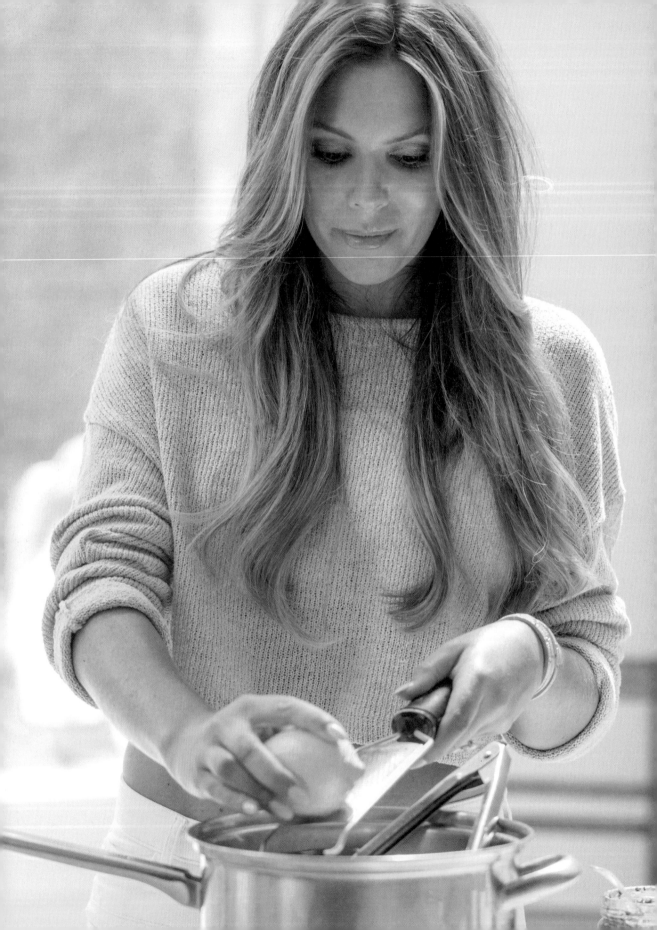

Getting fit and healthy is not just about exercise; what you eat and how you fuel your body is also hugely important. A balanced diet is one that provides you with all the energy and nutrients you need for an active life. The more you move, the more you can eat – a simple equation that motivates me every day! I've also learnt that a healthy diet shouldn't be viewed as a quick fix but more as a way to live your life, by eating a variety of wholesome foods that you can enjoy with family and friends.

eat

These days I think I actually eat more than I have ever done. What has changed is that I eat different foods and follow a balanced diet, plus I exercise more, which in turn gives me a healthy appetite. It's a combination that works for me – I don't deprive myself of one particular food group and I eat to feel full. It's something that I still have to work at but it's an approach to food that helps me to maintain a healthy weight.

Years ago my first instinct whenever I was unhappy with my weight or general health was to try to eat very little. It never worked – eventually your body and mind fight back and you get so hungry that you finally snap and wolf down something you really shouldn't. Then the guilt kicks in and, before you know it, you're on that emotional rollercoaster of self-denial and frustration.

Now I try to follow a more sensible diet that fills me up and is rich in vegetables and plant-based foods, lean proteins, complex carbohydrates and healthy fats. I usually have some kind of protein source at most main meals, avoid processed foods and favour complex carbs over simple carbohydrates. (Simple carbs, such as sugar and white breads, are easily digested and raise glucose levels quickly, while complex carbs found in wholegrains, vegetables, fruits and berries are more nutritious and release energy more slowly.)

I also try to keep my diet varied – it's really easy to get stuck in a rut, as with exercise. And it's important to enjoy your food – just like exercise again – so I try to pack in lots of delicious foods, such as avocados, fish, toasted nuts and seeds, so that I really look forward to meal times. Every now and then I will

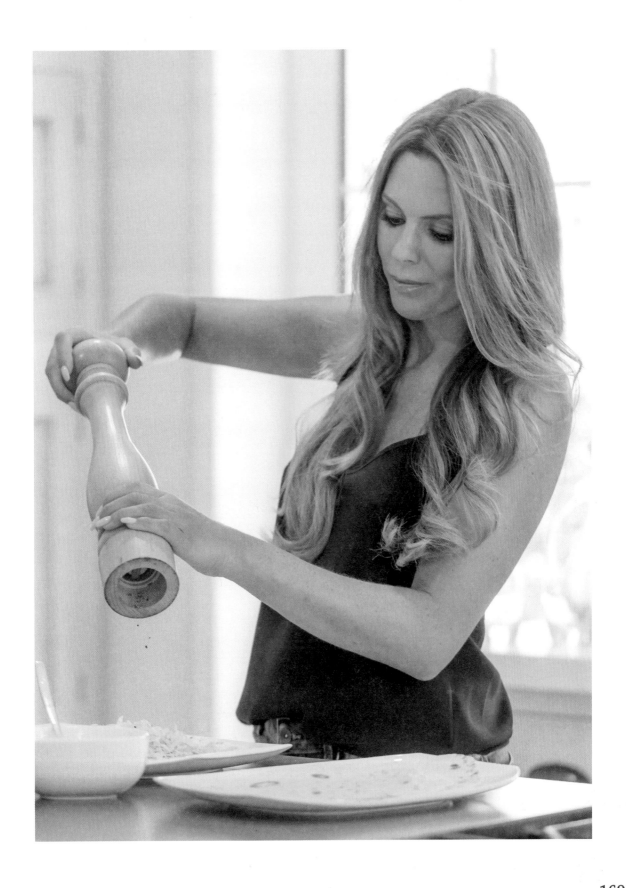

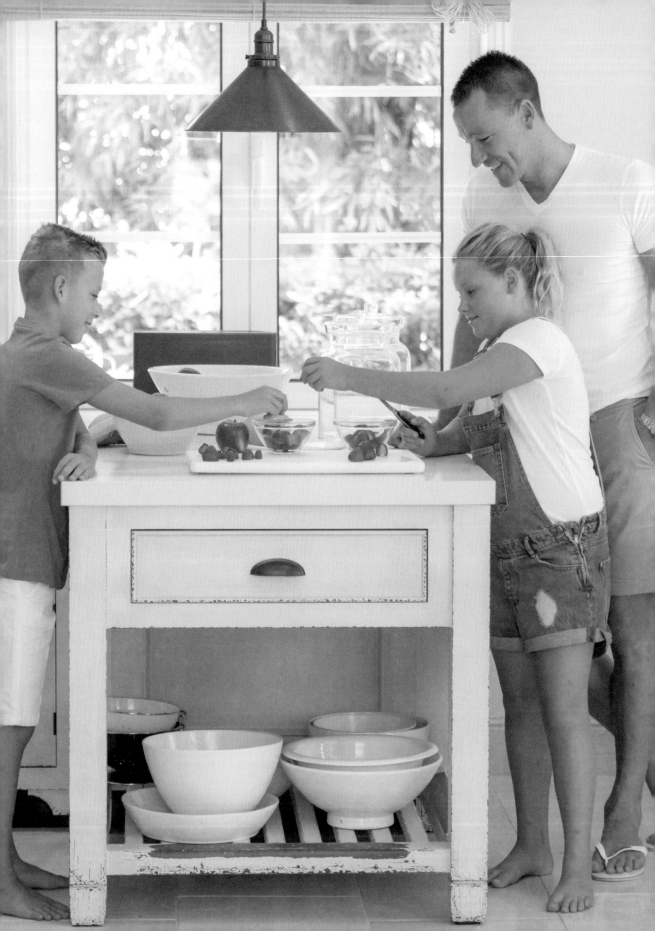

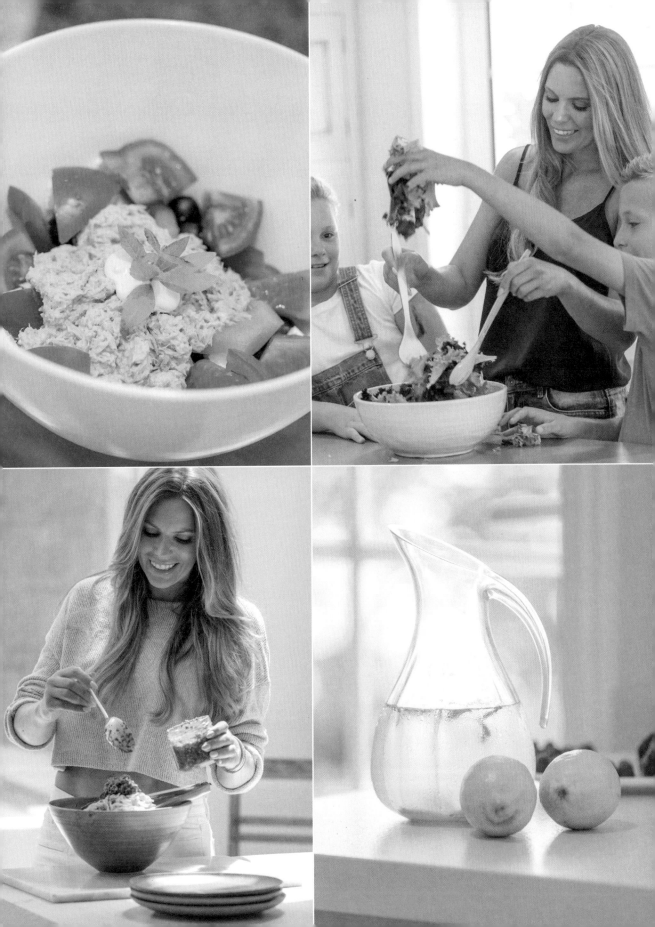

eat something I shouldn't – we're all human and when you're cooking for, or eating with, family or friends you do occasionally go off-piste. The key is to strike a balance: if you eat a slice or two of pizza one evening, then follow it up with a really healthy breakfast and a good workout the next morning.

When it comes to what to eat before or after working out, my advice is to figure out what works for you. I tend to work out in the morning without eating (that is 'train fasted'), and will then refuel afterwards. Other people have to eat at least 60 minutes before working out to keep their energy levels up. If you do eat a meal before a workout, it's usually best to do so a couple of hours before to allow your stomach to settle. After exercise, it's good to have a combination of good-quality protein to help with the recovery of muscle and carbohydrates as they'll replenish glycogen stores that may have become depleted after a workout and provide you with energy.

Maintaining a healthy diet isn't always easy – you do need to stay focused and be aware of what you're putting into your body. Think about what you're eating.

The recipes in this book aim to provide a combination of healthy nutrients, will keep you fuelled up during the day and are all dishes I love to cook and eat. Some of the meals or snacks can be prepared in advance and are perfect for meals on the go or packed lunches. There are some nutritious snacks, healthy dishes to share with your buddies, as well as some old family favourites, which are always a winner in the Terry household. I'll often get the kids involved in preparing the food as it's good for them to see what goes into their meals, and they enjoy cooking (particularly the chocolate brownies!). These recipes don't aim to cut out single food groups, such as carbs or dairy, as most of us have no need to avoid these totally but I have indicated occasionally which recipes are gluten-free.

Maintaining a healthy diet isn't always easy – you do need to stay focused and be aware of what you're putting into your body. Think about what you're eating – don't eat in front of the television or rush your food – and try to savour food and listen to your body. Just like an exercise programme, you'll have ups and downs but the key is to think positively, get your buddies involved and share ideas with them, and discover new and healthy foods along the way.

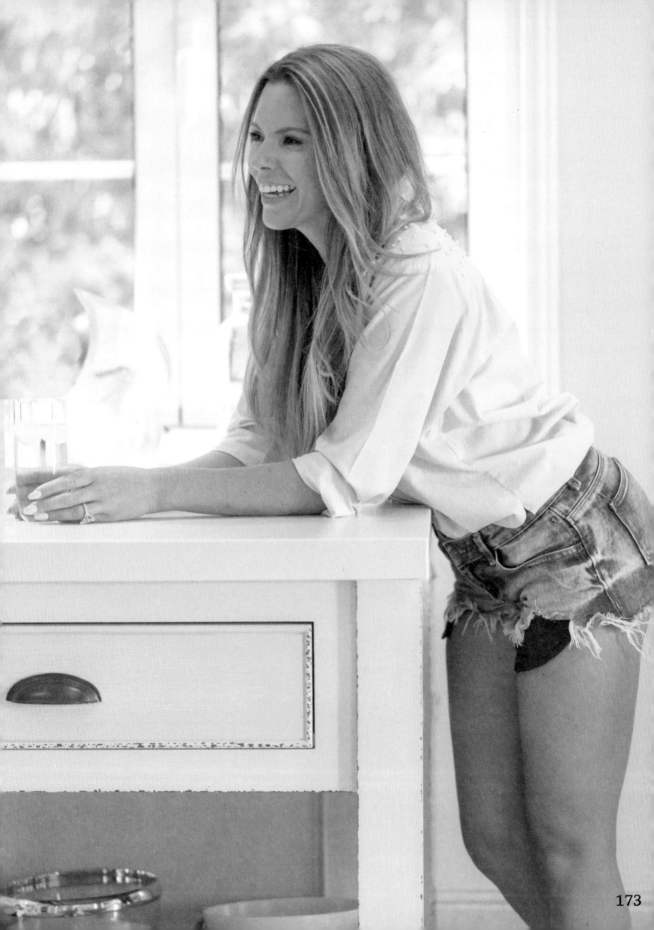

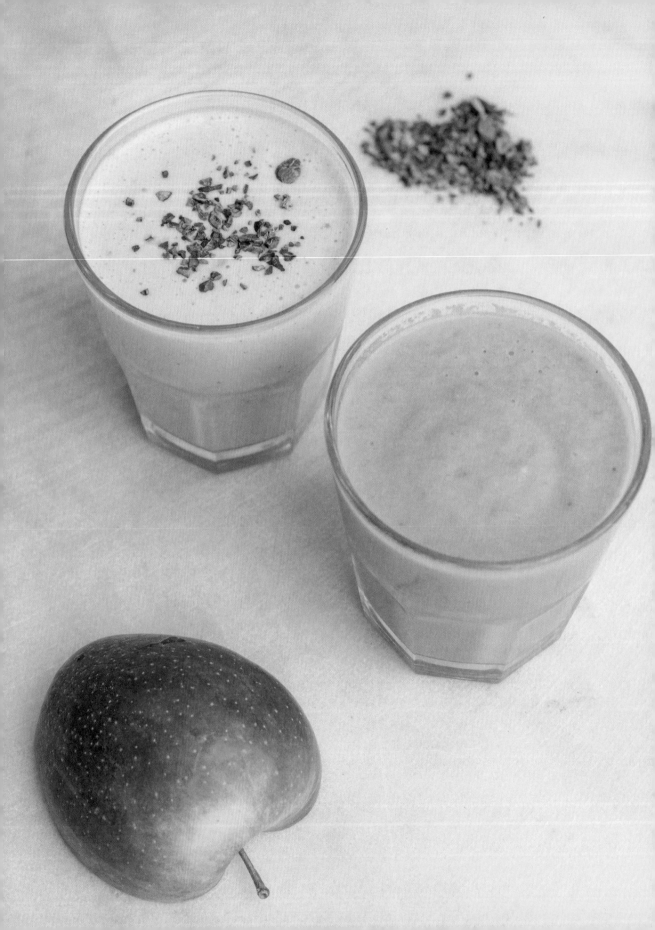

breakfast

apple and sultana oats

The oats in this breakfast can fuel
a workout or slowly release energy
throughout the day. You can soak
the oats overnight or for just half
an hour before breakfast.

90 g/3 oz porridge oats
180 ml/6 fl. oz almond milk
180 ml/6 fl. oz cloudy apple juice
plus 2 tablespoons
1 tablespoon sultanas
Half an apple, cored and sliced
Small handful of seeds such as
pumpkin, sunflower, linseed
Small handful of whole almonds

SERVES 1

Put the oats in a bowl, pour over the
almond milk and 180 ml/6 fl. oz
apple juice and stir. Set aside for
30 minutes. Combine the sultanas
with the extra 2 tablespoons of the
apple juice and leave for 30 minutes.

If soaking the night before, transfer
the oats and sultanas to sealed
containers and put in the fridge.

When you're ready to eat the
porridge, top with slices of apple, the
soaked sultanas, seeds and almonds.

TIP – *You could top these oats with any topping of
your choice, or soak them in orange juice instead of
apple juice.*

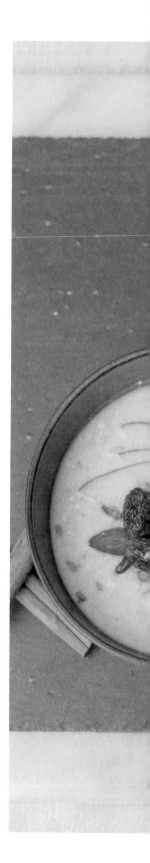

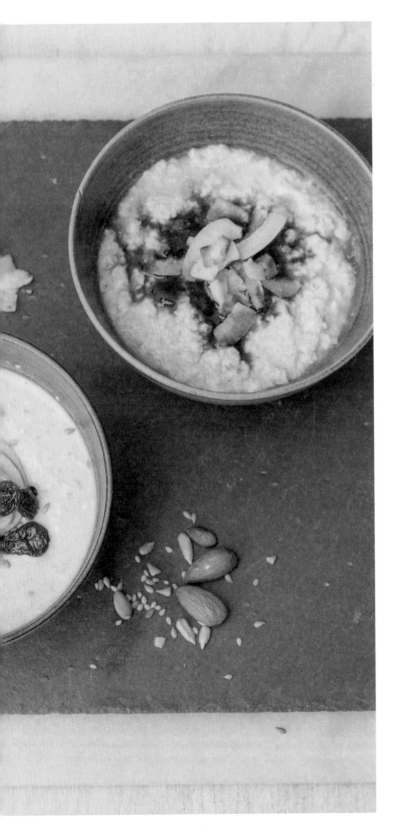

coconut and cinnamon oats

Coconut milk is packed with healthy vitamins and minerals and when added to oats makes for a creamy, energy-giving porridge.

90 g/3 oz porridge oats
375 ml–500 ml/12–16 fl. oz coconut milk
Pinch of cinnamon
Cocoa nibs (available in good health food shops)
Coconut shavings
Coconut yoghurt

SERVES 1

Combine the oats with the coconut milk. Set aside to soak for 30 minutes or transfer to a sealed container and leave in the fridge overnight.

Sprinkle on the cinnamon, top with cocoa nibs, coconut shavings and coconut yoghurt.

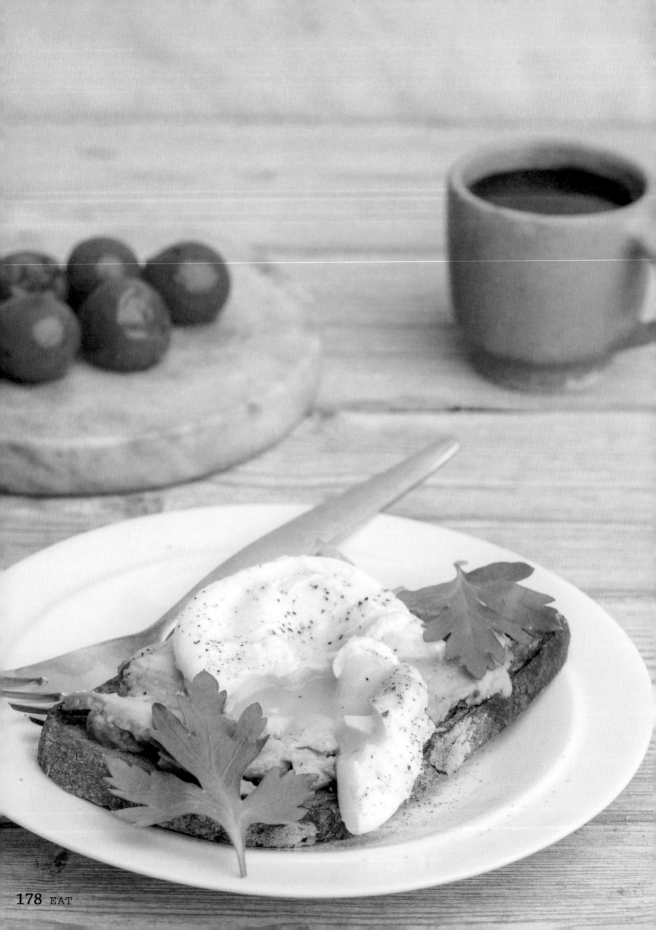

avocado on toast with a poached egg

Toast doesn't have to be boring, and a soft egg with toasted sourdough and avocado is my idea of heaven! This breakfast provides good-quality protein, nutritious and healthy fats and slow-releasing energy.

1 tablespoon cider vinegar
1 egg
1 slice sourdough bread
Half an avocado, destoned
1 tablespoon good olive oil
Salt and black pepper
Cherry tomatoes and parsley to serve (optional)

SERVES 1

Bring a small saucepan of water to the boil, then add the vinegar. Crack the egg into the boiling water and it will almost instantly form into a white ball. Simmer for 2–3 minutes.

In the meantime, toast your sourdough bread under a grill or in a toaster. Slice or mash the avocado and season with salt and pepper.

Drizzle the toast with most of the olive oil, then add the avocado. Remove the egg from the water with a slotted spoon, and put it on top of the toast. Add salt and pepper and a splash of olive oil. Serve with a few cherry tomatoes and parsley.

buckwheat pancakes

These pancakes are filling, nutritious and gluten-free. Even better, they're easy to make and delicious with honey and yoghurt or any topping of your choice.

FOR THE PANCAKES:
300 ml/10 ½ fl. oz almond milk
1 tablespoon yoghurt
1 tablespoon honey
Zest of 1 lemon or orange
225 g/8 oz buckwheat flour
1 teaspoon baking powder
Half a teaspoon cinnamon
1 large egg
1 teaspoon coconut oil, rapeseed oil or a knob of butter

FOR THE TOPPING:
Greek yoghurt
Fresh berries
Honey or maple syrup to drizzle

MAKES 6 FAT PANCAKES

Mix together the almond milk, yoghurt, honey and zest in a large bowl.

Combine the buckwheat flour, baking powder and cinnamon in another large bowl. Make a well in the centre of the flour, crack the egg into the well and gently pour the milk mixture over the egg.

Whisk gently using an electric whisk or a hand-held one, slowly incorporating the dry mixture into the wet mixture.

Heat a non-stick frying pan and add a small knob of the oil or butter. When the pan is hot, use a ladle or large serving spoon to spoon in the mixture, covering the bottom of the pan. Cook the first side for 1–2 minutes until it starts to bubble up around the edges and on top. Flip over onto the other side and continue to cook until speckled and golden. Remove from the pan, lay on a warm plate and repeat until you have six pancakes.

Serve the pancakes topped with fresh berries and a big spoon of Greek yoghurt. Drizzle with honey or maple syrup.

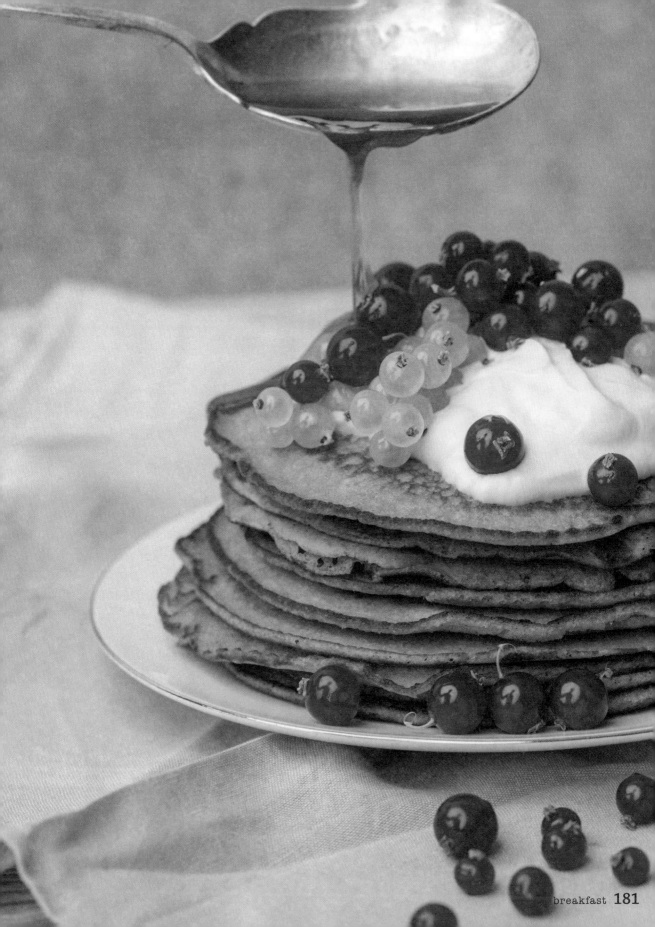

protein shakes

These fresh and vibrant shakes are quick to make, packed with nutrients and are perfect after a workout to aid recovery and provide energy for the rest of the day.

zingy green shake

Handful of baby spinach or kale
1 apple, cored and cut into quarters
Half a banana
Juice of half a lemon
Quarter of an avocado
20–30 g/½–1 oz fresh ginger, depending how you like it
1 tablespoon oats
1 tablespoon coconut oil (melted)
1 teaspoon hemp powder
150–200 ml/5–7 fl. oz made up of 50/50 apple juice and water

MAKES 2 MEDIUM GLASSES

Put all the ingredients in a blender or liquidizer and whiz up until you have a smooth consistency.

banana shake

1 banana
180 ml/6 fl. oz low-fat yoghurt
100 ml/3 ½ fl. oz almond milk or water
1 tablespoon oats
2 teaspoon protein or whey powder
1 teaspoon cinnamon
1 tablespoon cocoa powder (optional)
1 teaspoon coconut oil
1 teaspoon honey (to sweeten, optional)
1 teaspoon cocoa nibs (available from good health food shops)

MAKES 2 MEDIUM GLASSES

Put all the ingredients in a blender or liquidizer and whiz up until you have a smooth consistency. Sprinkle with cocoa nibs.

TIP – *You could replace the cocoa powder with any kind of berry, such as raspberries or blueberries.*

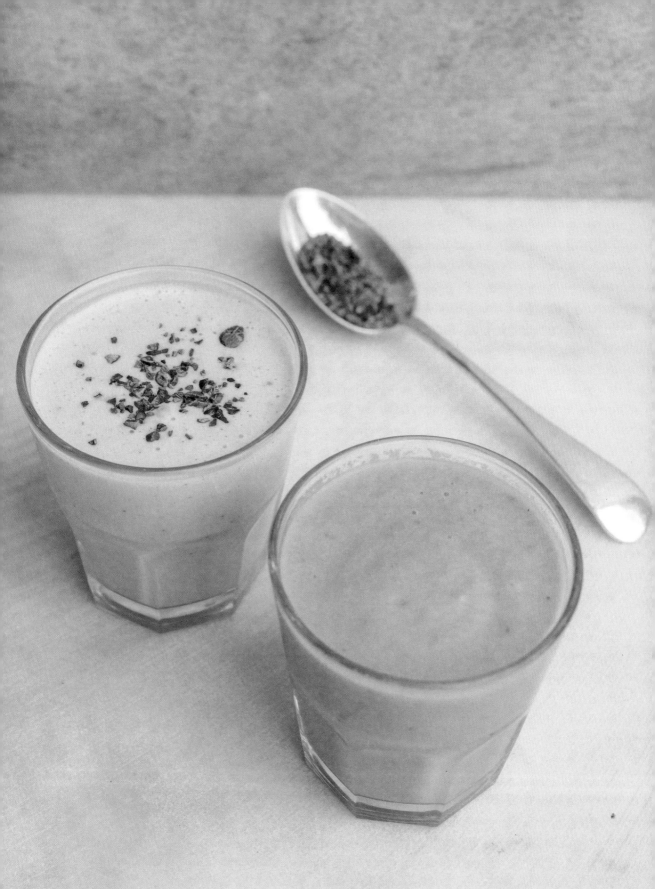

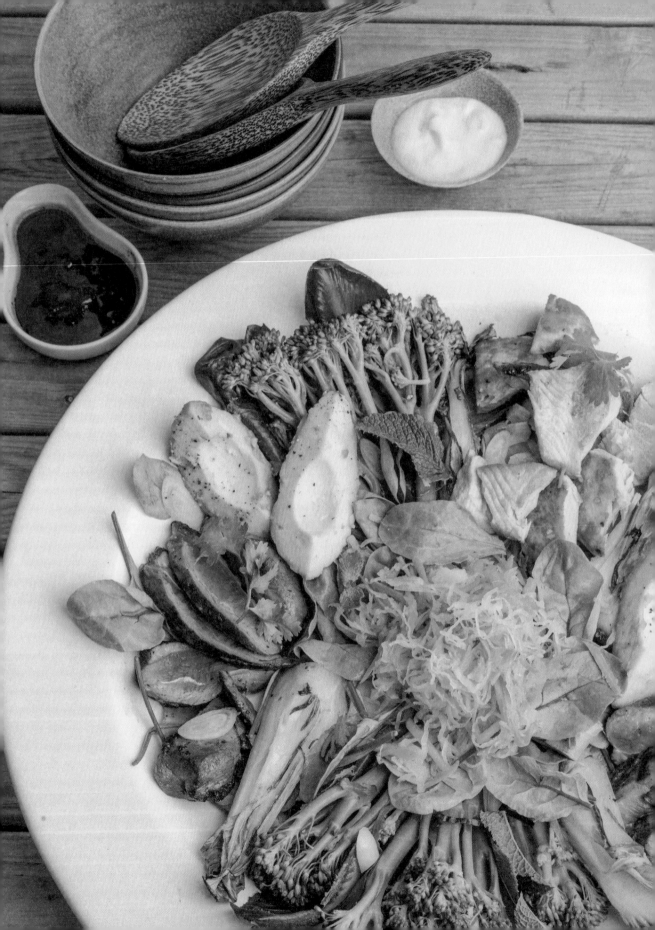

lunch

roasted red pepper and fresh tomato soup

This vibrantly coloured soup is packed with flavour and my children adore it. It's really warming and, during the winter months, it brightens even the coldest of days. In the summer, it can also be eaten as a chilled soup.

2 red peppers, halved and seeded
12 fresh tomatoes on the vine
2 garlic cloves, whole
3 tablespoons olive oil
1 onion, diced
1 celery stick, diced
550 ml/1 pint chicken stock
Salt and black pepper

TO SERVE:
150 ml/5 fl. oz sour cream
Fresh parsley, roughly chopped

SERVES 4-6

Grill the red peppers, tomatoes and garlic for 15–20 minutes until they get some colour, allowing the peppers to turn a little black so you can peel them. Peel the peppers and garlic cloves when cooled.

Put 1–2 tablespoons of the olive oil in a medium saucepan, add the onion and celery and cook until softened. Add the peeled peppers, tomatoes and peeled garlic. Pour in the chicken stock and simmer for 30 minutes, adding salt and pepper as needed.

Remove from the heat, then blitz with a hand blender until smooth. To serve, add some sour cream and olive oil, and sprinkle with parsley.

TIP – *You could make batches of this soup in late summer when tomatoes are at their ripest and store in the freezer.*

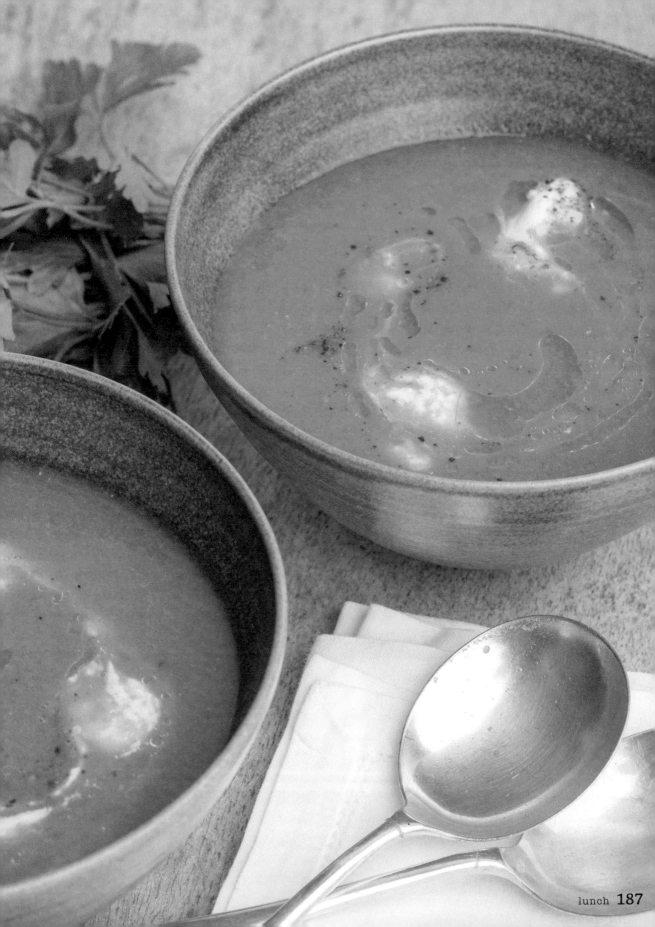

chicken skewers with quinoa salad

This makes for a great lunch. Quinoa is gluten-free and high in protein, the feta gives a tangy flavour and the hazelnuts add a bit of nutritious crunch. Yum!

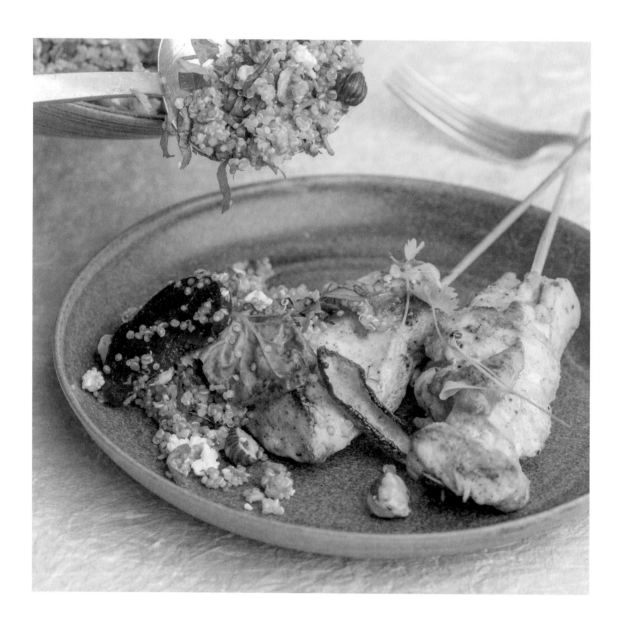

FOR THE CHICKEN:

4–5 free range, organic chicken breasts, diced
2 sprigs of thyme, chopped
Squeeze of lemon
Splash of olive oil
Generous sprinkle of turmeric powder
Salt and black pepper

FOR THE SALAD:

180 g/6 oz quinoa
Lemon zest
Splash of olive oil
750 ml–1 l/1½ –2 pints chicken stock
Half a red onion, thinly sliced
4 tablespoons good red wine vinegar
2 teaspoons brown sugar
Handful of spinach
1 pack of 4 cooked beetroots
Half a bunch of coriander
Half a bunch of parsley
100 g/3½ oz hazelnuts, roughly chopped
100 g/3½ oz crumbled feta
Salt and black pepper

FOR THE DRESSING:

Juice of 3–4 lemons
Juice of 4 limes
125ml/4 fl. oz cider vinegar
2 tablespoons honey
Salt and black pepper

SERVES 4

Combine the chicken, thyme, lemon juice and seasoning with a splash of olive oil and turmeric in a bowl and leave for half an hour. Preheat the oven to 180°C/350°F.

Put the quinoa in a saucepan with the lemon zest, seasoning and olive oil. Cook without any liquid for 2 minutes on a low heat, giving the pan a shake before pouring over the stock. Place a lid on the saucepan and continue to cook for around 10–12 minutes. Most of the liquid should be absorbed and the quinoa will look puffed up.

Turn the heat off and leave the lid on the saucepan for 5–10 minutes.

Put the sliced red onion in a bowl with the red wine vinegar and sugar. Set aside for 20 minutes.

Add the spinach while the quinoa is still warm, as well as the beetroot (chopped as fine or as chunky at you like), chopped herbs, hazelnuts, red onion and crumbled feta.

Thread the chicken onto skewers. This should make four. Get a frying pan nice and hot and seal the chicken pieces on both sides, giving them a golden colour. This should take 2–3 minutes on each side. Place in the oven for 10–12 minutes.

For the dressing, combine the lemon and lime juice, cider vinegar, honey and seasoning. Pour over the chicken and serve alongside the quinoa salad.

TIP - *Raw onion in salad can sometimes have a pungent aftertaste, which can be prevented by soaking it in vinegar and sugar.*

rice salad with peas and herbs

I love this gluten-free vegetarian salad. The rice
is full of slow-release energy and chickpeas are
a good source of protein – and it tastes good too.

Half a red onion, thinly sliced
2–3 tablespoons lemon juice
Half a teaspoon of sugar
45 g/1½ oz brown rice and
wild rice mix
2 handfuls of frozen peas
1 small broccoli, broken into florets
120 g/4 oz tinned chickpeas or
black eyed beans
1 small celery stick, diced
Handful of spinach
Half a small bunch of mint,
roughly chopped
Half a small bunch of coriander,
roughly chopped
Salt and black pepper

SERVES 4

Put the red onion in a bowl with the lemon juice and
sugar and leave to one side for 30 minutes. (This pickles
the onion and takes away the rawness.)

Put the rice and 500ml/16 fl. oz of water in a saucepan,
bring to the boil and then simmer over a low heat for
20 minutes until the water is absorbed. Take off the heat,
add the frozen peas while the rice is still warm and leave
to stand for 5 minutes.

Bring a saucepan of water to the boil, add the broccoli and
cook for 3 minutes. Drain and add to the rice.

Add the chickpeas, celery, spinach and the onion with a
little of the lemon juice. Mix in the mint and coriander,
season and serve.

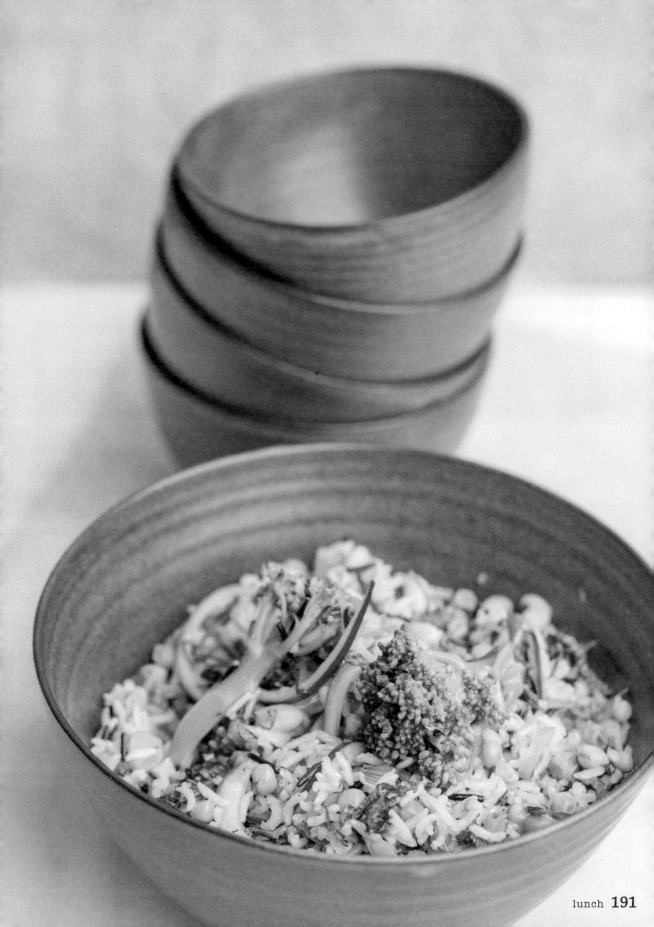

sweet potato, cherry tomato and spinach frittata

This is a great lunchtime dish – it's nutritious with good-quality protein, easy to make and, with the soft roasted sweet potato, tastes incredible.

400 g/14 oz (around 2) sweet potatoes, peeled and cut into chunks
5 tablespoons olive oil
1 teaspoon fresh thyme, chopped
10–12 cherry tomatoes
150 g/5 oz spinach
6 eggs
Small bunch of parsley, chopped
Salt and black pepper
Green salad, to serve

SERVES 6-8

Preheat the oven to 180°C/350°F. Put the sweet potato on a non-stick baking tray with 2 tablespoons of the olive oil, the thyme, salt and pepper, and bake for 20 minutes. After 10 minutes, add the cherry tomatoes to the tray.

In a medium-sized frying pan, cook the spinach with 1 tablespoon of oil for 1 minute until it wilts. Remove the spinach and put in a bowl (as you will use the frying pan for the frittata).

Take the sweet potatoes and tomatoes out of the oven, set aside and increase the heat to 200°C/390°F.

Put the medium-sized frying pan back on a medium heat, adding the rest of the olive oil (1–2 tablespoons). In a bowl, whisk the eggs with the salt and pepper. Mix in the potatoes, tomatoes and chopped parsley, and pour into the hot frying pan. Arrange the wilted spinach on top.

Cook the egg mixture for 2–3 minutes until it starts bubbling. Then put the pan in the oven and bake for 15–20 minutes. Serve with a green salad.

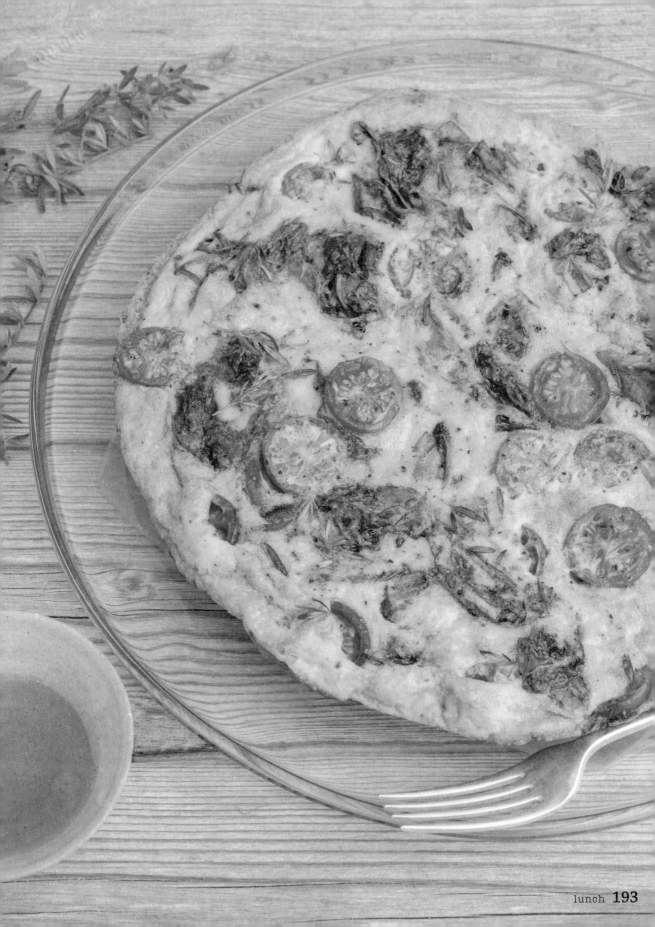

wholemeal wraps

Wraps are the perfect grab-and-go lunch but sometimes they need a little jazzing up to make them interesting. These two options are positively bursting with nutrition and flavour.

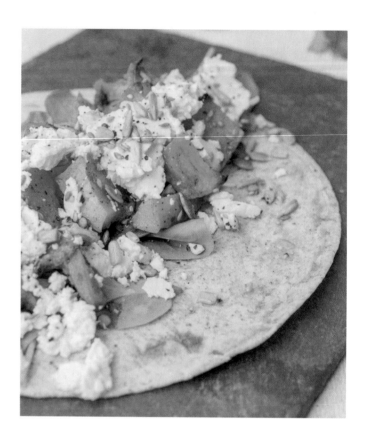

squash and feta wrap

400 g/14 oz squash, peeled and cut into large chunks
2 sprigs of thyme, chopped
2 tablespoons olive oil
2 wholemeal wraps
150 g/5 oz feta cheese
Handful of spinach
Handful of coriander
Handful of toasted seeds
Salt and black pepper

MAKES 2 GENEROUS WRAPS

Preheat the oven to 180°C/350°F.

Mix the squash and fresh thyme with the oil and salt and pepper in a baking dish and roast in the oven for 30 minutes.

Remove the squash from the oven and place on the wraps. Add the feta, spinach, coriander and seeds. Roll up the wrap and devour!

salmon and rocket wrap

120 g/4 oz frozen peas
1 tablespoon olive oil
2 tablespoons yoghurt
2 wholemeal wraps
120–150 g/4–5 oz smoked salmon
1 avocado, destoned and sliced
Handful of rocket
Handful of mint leaves
Salt and black pepper

MAKES 2 GENEROUS WRAPS

Put the frozen peas in a small saucepan with the olive oil and 1–2 tablespoons of water, salt and pepper. Cook for 2–3 minutes over a medium–high heat.

Remove the peas from the heat, and using a potato masher, roughly crush them. Stir in the yoghurt and season to taste.

Smear a dollop of peas across the middle of the wraps, pull the salmon into long strips and place on top, then add the avocado, a handful of rocket and mint leaves, season and roll up.

TIP - *A good, gluten-free alternative to wholemeal wraps are quinoa or chia seed wraps, which are available in good health food stores.*

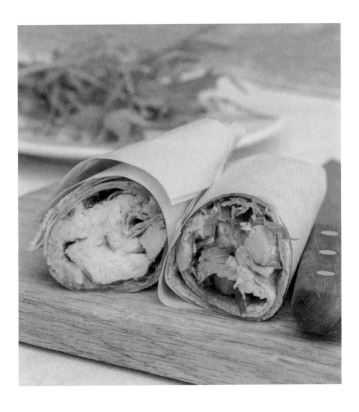

king prawns with cucumber, carrots and edamame bean salad

This Asian-inspired salad has just a little bit of a kick to it – and is packed full of crunchy, fresh veggies.

FOR THE SALAD:
220 g/8 oz raw king prawns
1 lemon
1 tablespoon olive oil
150 g/5 oz pack bean sprouts
Half a cucumber, deseeded
1 red pepper, deseeded
1 carrot, peeled
Handful of edamame beans
Handful of baby spinach
Half a bunch of fresh mint, leaves picked
Half a bunch of fresh coriander
1 tablespoon plain peanuts, (optional)
Salt and black pepper

FOR THE DRESSING:
60 ml/2 fl. oz lime juice
1 red chilli, deseeded and finely chopped
1 garlic clove, crushed
Half a teaspoon brown sugar
1 tablespoon honey
2 tablespoons fish sauce
2 tablespoons good vegetable or rapeseed oil

SERVES 2

Put the prawns in a small bowl, season and add a squeeze of lemon with a little zest, and the olive oil. Fry the prawns in a hot pan over a high heat. Toss for 2–3 minutes until they turn pink. Leave to one side.

Soak the bean sprouts in water for 10 minutes and then drain. Set aside.

Cut the deseeded cucumber, pepper and carrot into thin sticks.

Heat a saucepan of water until boiling, add the edamame beans and cook over a high heat for 3–4 minutes. Drain and set aside.

Put the carrot, cucumber, pepper, bean sprouts and edamame beans in a bowl. Add the spinach, mint and coriander, leaving some of the stalks on the coriander.

Toast the peanuts in a small frying pan over a medium heat for 2–3 minutes until they brown slightly.

For the dressing, put the lime juice, chilli, garlic, sugar, honey, fish sauce and oil in a small bowl. Mix and season. Pour over the salad and toss, adding the prawns last. Scatter over the toasted peanuts.

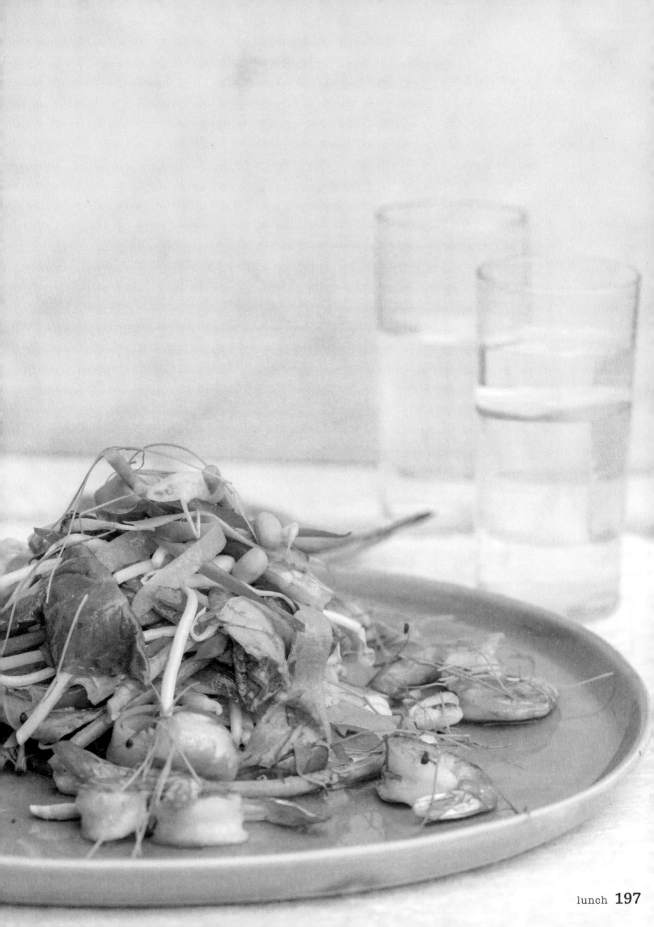

buddy bowl

If you have some buddies coming round, serve up this large dish of nutritious goodies and let your friends create their own buddy bowl. This version has a variety of interesting Asian-inspired toppings and two types of dressing.

Preheat the oven to 180°C/350°F. In a bowl, combine the carrot with the sauerkraut. Mix together the vinegar, the sugar and 2 tablespoons of the oil with some salt and pepper and pour over the carrot mix. Set aside.

Put the salmon on a baking tray, add some lemon zest and a squeeze of juice along with 1 tablespoon of the rapeseed oil and bake in the oven for 5–6 minutes.

If using the duck breasts, trim off some of the fat around the edges. Then lightly score the remaining fat crossways over the breast. Drizzle with honey and salt and pepper. Heat 2 teaspoons of oil in a frying pan until hot, place the duck skin-side down in the pan and fry for 5 minutes over a medium heat until the skin is nicely golden. Turn and cook for another 3 minutes. Put to one side to rest. Bring a medium-sized saucepan with water

to the boil. Cut the bok choy down the middle and add it and the broccoli to the pan. Cook for 2 minutes. Drain and season the vegetables, and add 1 tablespoon of oil.

Slice the duck, flake the fish and break up the chicory leaf. Arrange on a platter or large plate with the broccoli and bok choy and add the avocado. Drizzle with the rest of the lemon juice. Scatter over the seaweed, pickled ginger, chilli, mint and coriander, and toasted seeds.

Make the two dressings by mixing all the ingredients together, and then put them in two small dishes.

TIP – *You can always replace the duck with another fish or more salmon. If you're vegetarian, replace the fish and meat with protein-rich lentils, tofu or cheese. If you want a complex carbohydrate, add steamed brown rice.*

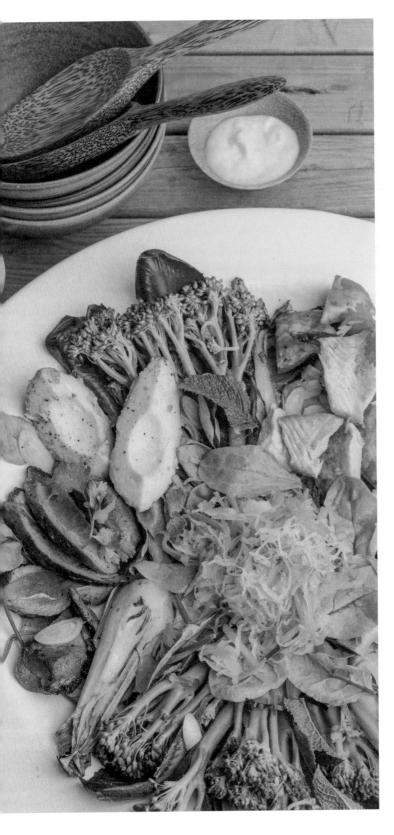

200 g/7 oz carrot, grated

100 g/3½ oz sauerkraut (available in most supermarkets)

1 tablespoon cider vinegar

1 tablespoon brown sugar

4–5 tablespoons good vegetable oil or rapeseed oil

2 x 140 g/5 oz salmon fillets (280 g/10 oz in total)

Juice and zest of 1 lemon

2 x 125 g/4½ oz duck breasts (250 g/9 oz in total) (optional)

2 teaspoons honey

250 g/9 oz bok choy

150 g/5 oz tender stem broccoli

1 red chicory, broken up (optional)

1 ripe avocado, destoned and sliced

FOR THE TOPPING:

Handful of seaweed strips (optional)

2 tablespoons pickled ginger (available in Asian stores and most supermarkets), roughly chopped

2 red chillies, deseeded, finely chopped

Half a bunch of mint, roughly torn

1 small bunch of coriander, roughly torn

Handful of mixed toasted seeds

FOR THE WASABI MAYO DRESSING:

4–5 tablespoons mayonnaise

Quarter to half a teaspoon of wasabi (depending on how hot you like it)

FOR THE GINGER SOYA DRESSING:

6 tablespoons soy sauce

1 tablespoon pickled ginger, roughly chopped (as above) and a little of the ginger juice, around 1–2 teaspoons

2 tablespoons sesame oil

SERVES 4

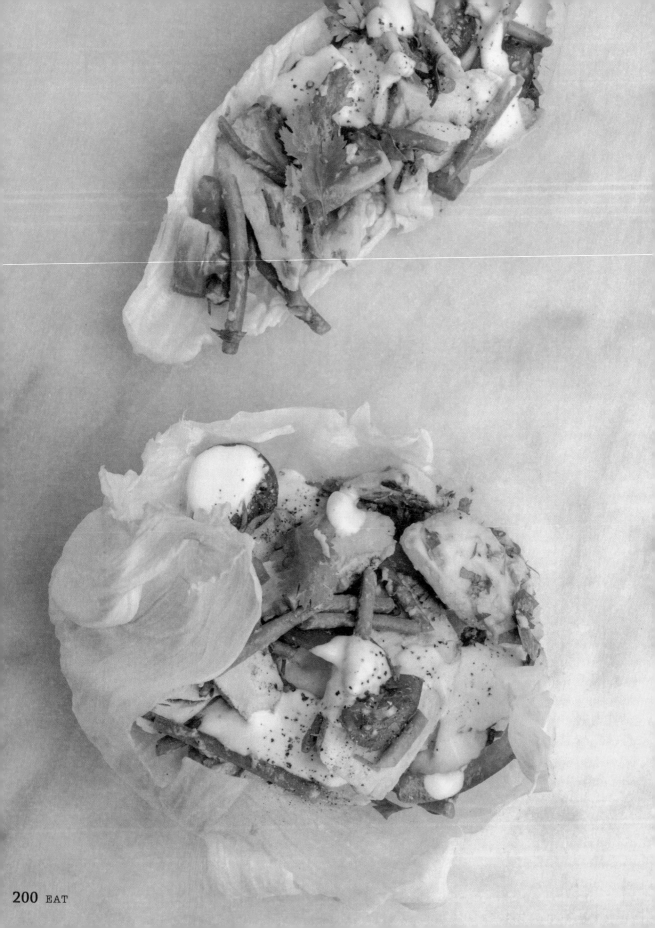

chicken and avocado lettuce wrap

These chicken parcels make for a light and really delicious lunch. The avocado is rich in healthy fats and you could also add a drop of Tabasco if you want a little zing!

2 teaspoons fresh thyme, chopped
1 teaspoon paprika
Zest and juice of 1 lemon
3 tablespoons olive oil
3 chicken breasts
110 g/4 oz green beans
Handful of parsley
Handful of coriander
2 avocados, halved and destoned
1–2 tablespoons mayonnaise
1 round lettuce, cos or iceberg
8–10 cherry tomatoes, halved
Tabasco (optional)
Salt and black pepper
Mayonnaise, to serve

SERVES 4

Mix together the thyme, paprika, juice and zest of half the lemon, a splash of olive oil and season. Add the chicken breasts and marinate for 30 minutes to 1 hour.

Preheat the oven to 180°C/350°F. Heat a frying pan, add 2 tablespoons of olive oil and fry the chicken breasts for 2–3 minutes on each side. Once the chicken has a nice golden colour put it in the oven for 10 minutes.

Put the green beans in a saucepan of boiling water and cook for 2–3 minutes. In a bowl, chop the parsley, coriander and avocado and mix with the mayonnaise. Add a squeeze of lemon or tabasco to taste.

Slice the chicken and add it with the drained green beans to the avocado mixture. Open up the lettuce and place the chicken mixture on one or two leaves, topped with some halved cherry tomatoes. Drizzle on some mayonnaise. You can then either roll it up like a wrap or leave it as an open parcel.

mixed leaf tuna salad

This is a staple lunch dish for me. It's simple, nutritious and a great source of protein, and it's perfect for a packed lunch when you're on the go.

Half a red pepper, deseeded and sliced
Handful of cherry tomatoes, halved
Quarter of a cucumber, sliced
6 black olives, destoned and halved
Handful of mixed leaf, rocket or baby spinach
1 112 g/4 oz tin of good-quality tuna
Juice of half a lemon
2 tablespoons sour cream
Salt and black pepper

SERVES 1

In bowl or plastic container, combine the pepper, tomatoes, cucumber, olives and mixed salad leaves. Mix in the tuna, drizzle with the lemon juice and the sour cream, and add seasoning.

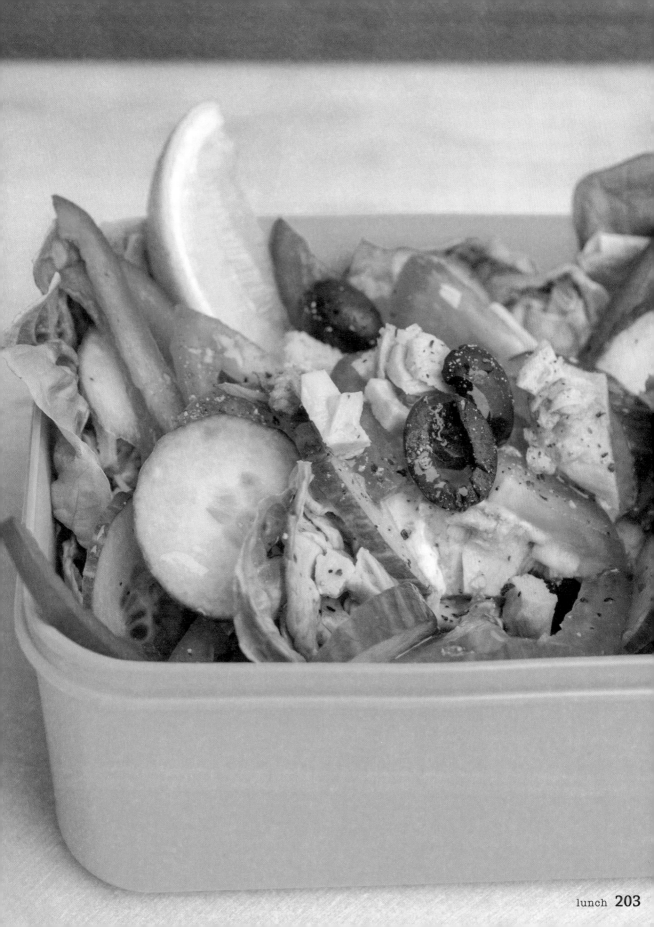

chicken satay with chunky carrot and cucumber salad

We all adore the nutty flavour of chicken satay and this also makes a great dish for friends. The salad of crunchy ribbons of carrots and cucumber can be made really quickly with a vegetable peeler.

4 skinless, boneless chicken breasts
1–2 tablespoons olive oil
Salt and black pepper

FOR THE SATAY SAUCE:

3 tablespoons dark or light soy sauce
1 tablespoon of chunky peanut butter
180 ml/6 fl. oz coconut milk
1 garlic clove, minced
Juice and zest of 2 limes
1 teaspoon mild curry powder
1 teaspoon ginger powder
A few drops of Tabasco

FOR THE SALAD:

2 carrots, peeled and cut into ribbons length-wise
1 cucumber, cut into ribbons length-wise
Handful of spinach
Juice of 1 lime
Splash of olive oil or sesame oil
Salt and black pepper
Coriander to serve

SERVES 4

Put all the satay sauce ingredients in a bowl and mix until combined.

Dice the chicken and add the seasoning. Mix in with the satay sauce and leave to marinate in the fridge for a couple of hours or overnight.

Using a frying pan with a lid, add 1–2 tablespoons of olive oil. Remove the chicken from the satay sauce and add it to the frying pan. Cook the chicken over a low heat, turning it regularly, for around 10 minutes. Put any remaining satay sauce in a small dish.

Make the salad by mixing up the ribbons of carrot and cucumber, spinach, lime juice, olive oil and seasoning. Serve with the satay sauce and chicken, and sprinkle the coriander on top.

TIP - *The satay sauce can be prepared in advance and put in the freezer.*

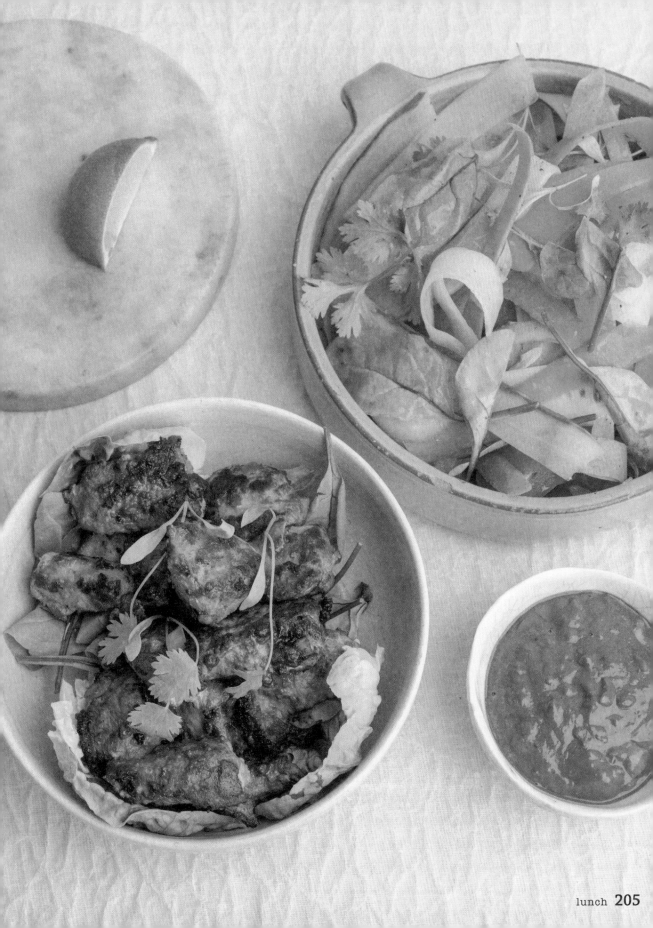

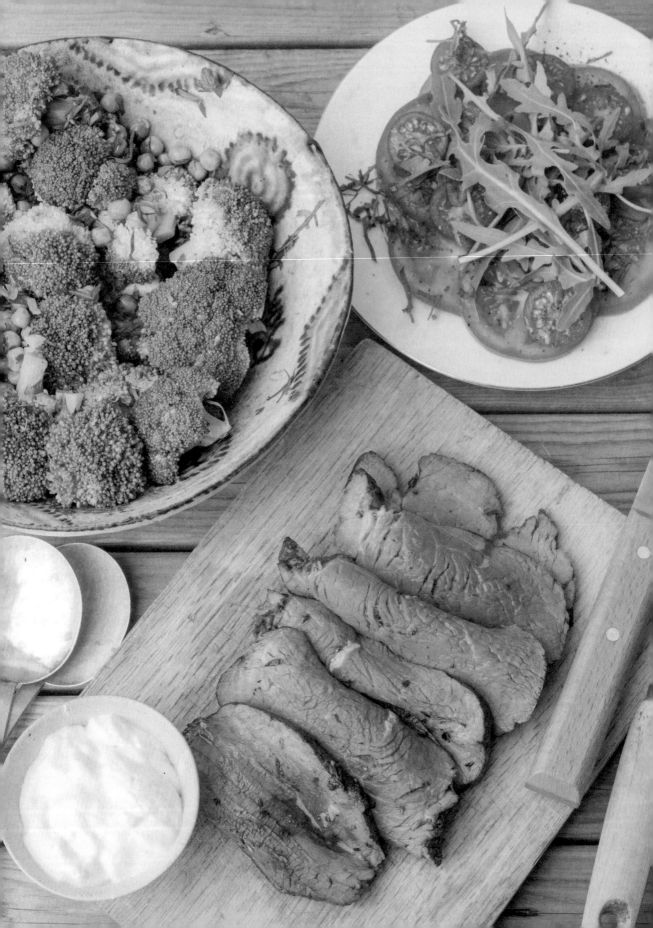

dinner

chicken burgers

My kids love burgers, but I know that these homemade versions are made with fresh and healthy ingredients. They can be eaten with or without the buns.

FOR THE BURGERS:

2 chicken breasts, minced (the butcher can do this, or blitz in a food processor at home)
Half a carrot, finely chopped
1 shallot
2 garlic cloves
3 chestnut mushrooms
5 cherry tomatoes, deseeded
Splash of olive oil
1 sprig of oregano
2 tablespoons plain flour or gluten-free cornmeal, plus a little extra for moulding the burgers
1 egg, beaten,
Salt and black pepper

TO SERVE:

4 wholemeal burger buns
Mayonnaise or tomato chutney
A bag of mixed leaf salad

MAKES 4 BURGERS

Preheat the oven to 180°C/350°F.

Put the chicken, carrot, shallot, garlic, mushrooms, tomatoes, oil, oregano, seasoning and 2 tablespoons of the flour in a food processor and mix until blended but not too smooth. When mixed, stir in a couple of spoonfuls of the beaten egg.

Scatter some flour or cornmeal on a plate and pat onto your hands. Mould the mixture into four round burger shapes.

Heat some oil in a frying pan over a medium–high heat, add the burgers and cook for 3–4 minutes each side until golden brown. Put the burgers in a roasting dish and cook in the oven for 10 minutes. Remove the burgers from the oven and cool for 1–2 minutes.

Cut open your buns and spread generously with mayonnaise and/or chutney. Pop your burgers in and serve with a mixed leaf salad.

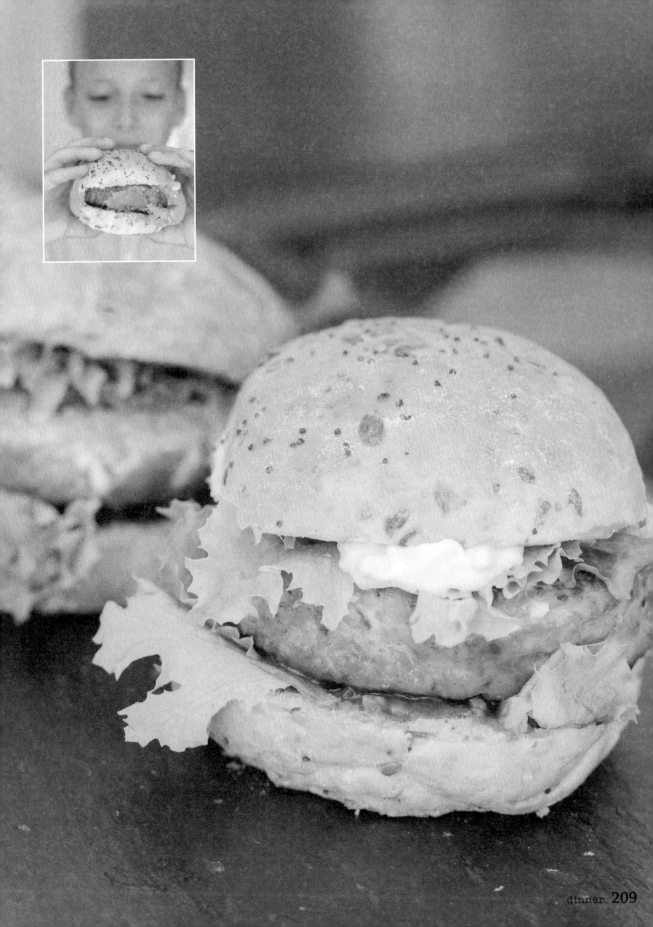

200 g/7 oz dried mushrooms
2 shallots, diced
2 garlic cloves, chopped
1 teaspoon fresh thyme
1 teaspoon fresh oregano
3–4 tablespoons olive oil
50 g/2 oz spelt (alternatively, replace
with risotto rice, spelt just makes the
risotto a bit lighter)
50 g/2 oz risotto rice
1 egg, beaten
2 tablespoons plain or polenta flour
Watercress or rocket salad, avocado
and squeeze of lime, to serve

SERVES 4–6

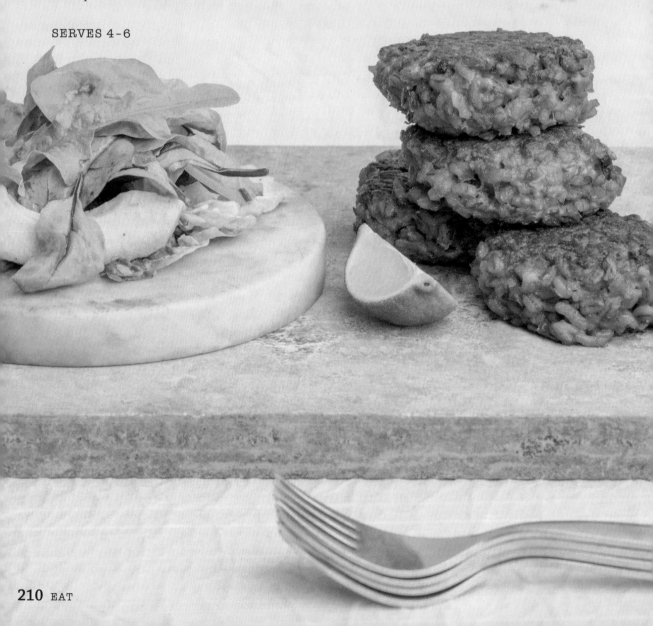

mushroom risotto cakes

These risotto cakes have a delicate mushroomy flavour and my family love them. You can also make them into smaller cakes, pop them in the fridge and use them for kids' packed lunches the next day.

Soak the dried mushrooms in 500–600ml/ 1–1½ pints boiled water. Set aside for 20 minutes.

Put the shallots, garlic, thyme and oregano in a saucepan with 1 tablespoon of the olive oil and cook over a medium heat for 5 minutes until soft. Add the spelt and rice and cook for 2 minutes, giving it a stir without adding any liquid. Now drain the mushrooms, reserving the water and adding it to the pan. (It looks like a lot of water but the rice will absorb it.)

Chop the softened mushrooms and add to the pan. Cook for around 45 minutes, keeping a careful eye on the risotto and stirring frequently, until the rice is soft and all the liquid has been absorbed.

Leave the rice to cool for half an hour. Stir in the beaten egg. Using your hands, mould the rice into 4–6 cakes, depending on how big you want them. Put the cakes in the fridge to chill for an hour before cooking.

Preheat the oven to 180°C/350°F. When the risotto cakes are chilled, scatter the polenta or plain flour on a plate and coat the cakes.

Heat 2–3 tablespoons of the olive oil in a frying pan over a medium heat. Add the cakes and fry them for 5–6 minutes on each side until crispy and golden.

Cook in the preheated oven for 10–15 minutes. Serve with a watercress or rocket salad, avocado and a squeeze of lime.

fresh herby pasta

Serve pasta with this super-simple pesto-like sauce that everyone will love. The sauce keeps well in the fridge so you can prepare it in advance and whip it out when you're short on time.

1 bunch of flat leaf parsley
Half a bunch of mint
1 garlic clove, sliced
1 teaspoon capers
125 ml/4 oz olive oil
125 ml/4 oz rapeseed oil
Zest of 1 lemon
500 g/1 lb tagliatelle or gluten-free pasta
Salt and black pepper

SERVES 4

Roughly remove the parsley leaves from the stalks. (It doesn't matter about some of the thinner stalks as they just add to the freshness.) Separate the mint leaves from their stalks.

Put the parsley, mint leaves, garlic, capers, olive oil and rapeseed oil in a blender and blitz. The sauce doesn't need to be super smooth so don't over-blend. Mix in the lemon zest.

Cook the pasta according to the packet instructions; usually 6–8 minutes.

Once cooked, drain the pasta and put in a big bowl, adding the green sauce while it's hot, and season.

TIP - *The sauce will keep in the fridge for 1–2 weeks if you cover the top with a little extra oil.*

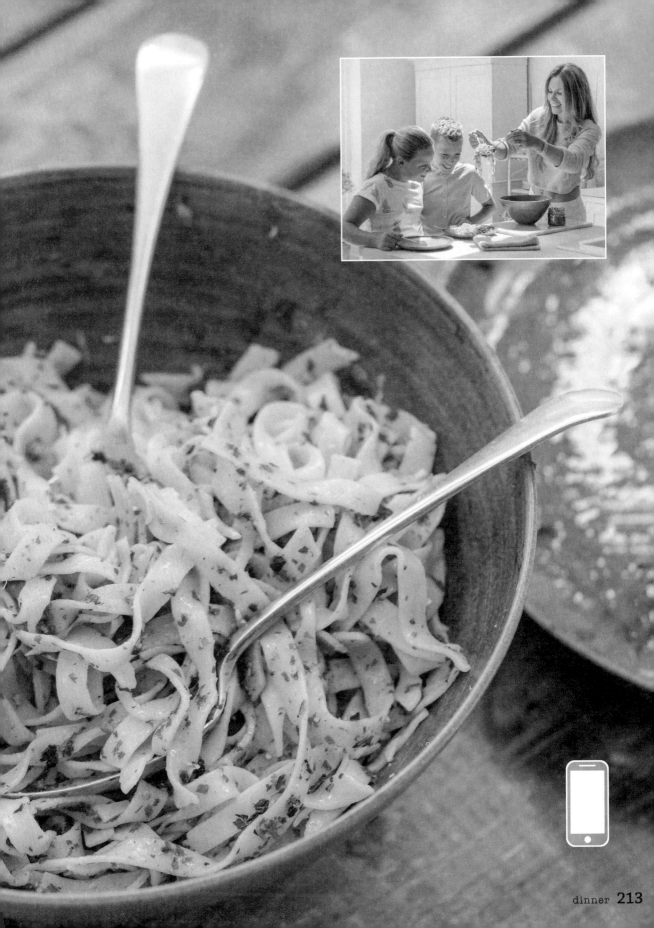

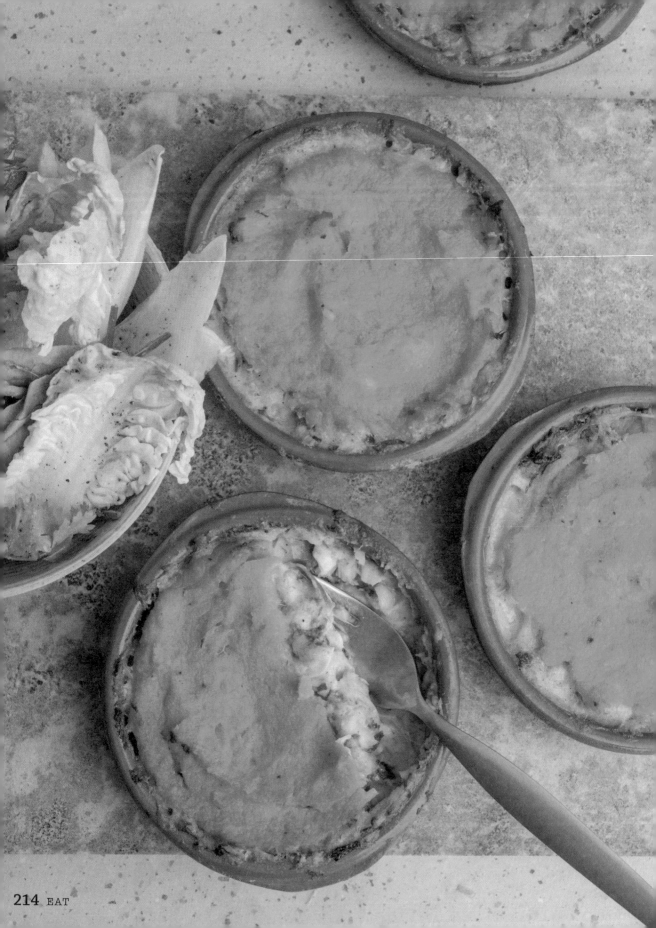

fish pies

There's nothing like coming home to fish pie after a long and exhausting day. Fish is of course high-protein and low-fat, and these pies are made with sweet potatoes which are more nutritious than regular potatoes. You can make this in individual small dishes or as one big dish.

450 g/1 lb cod
Juice and zest of 1 lime
1 teaspoon fennel seeds
2 large sweet potatoes, peeled and cut into chunks
1 leek, cut into chunks
120 g/4 oz butter
80–100 g/3–3½ oz spelt or plain flour
550 ml/1 pint semi-skimmed milk
Small bunch of parsley, chopped
Handful of tarragon, chopped
Splash of olive oil
Salt and black pepper
Green salad and slice of lemon, to serve

SERVES 4

TIP - *You could substitute the sweet potato topping for a variety of vegetables, such as celeriac or regular potatoes.*

Preheat the oven to 180°C/350°F.

Put the cod on a baking tray, add the lime zest and juice, fennel seeds, salt and pepper. Cover in foil and cook in the oven for 15 minutes or until flaky. Set aside.

Put the sweet potatoes in a saucepan, cover with water and bring to the boil. Reduce the heat and simmer for around 20 minutes or until soft.

Meanwhile, put the leek and the butter in a saucepan and cook for 5–6 minutes over a low heat until the leek has softened. Then add the flour and stir. Cook for 1–2 minutes and then slowly add the milk, stirring as you go. Cook for a further 4–5 minutes until the sauce starts to thicken.

Flake the cooked fish into the sauce. Then add the parsley and tarragon, stir and season. Put the fish mixture into small dishes or one big dish.

Drain the potatoes, add the olive oil, salt and pepper and mash them. Spread the mash over the fish mixture.

Cook in the oven for 25 minutes until the pie topping is bubbling and has a little colour. Serve with a green salad and a slice of lemon.

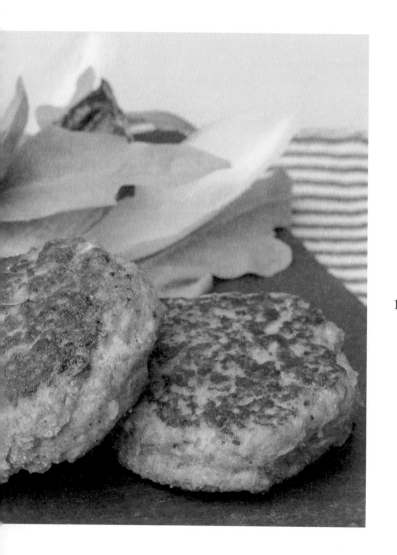

FOR THE FISH CAKES:

1 large potato, peeled and roughly diced
350 g/12 oz salmon fillet
Zest and juice of 1 lime
2–3 tablespoons olive oil
Half a bunch of parsley, chopped
Flour (for moulding)
Salt and black pepper
Squeeze of lemon to serve

FOR THE SAUCE

225 g/8 oz yoghurt
Zest of 1 lemon
1 tablespoon capers, roughly chopped
Half a bunch of coriander, chopped
Salt and black pepper

FOR THE SALAD:

1 bag of mixed salad leaves
Large fennel bulb, thinly sliced
Olive oil
Drizzle of balsamic vinegar

MAKES 4

fish cakes

Oily fish like salmon is a great high-quality protein, packed with vitamins and healthy omega-3 fats. These fish cakes come with a lovely creamy sauce and are just delicious.

Preheat the oven to 180°C/350°F. Heat a saucepan of water, add the potato pieces and boil for 15 minutes until soft.

Line a baking tray with greaseproof paper. Add the salmon, sprinkle on the lime zest and juice, and cook in the oven for 15 minutes.

Once the potato is cooked, mash with a splash of olive oil. Remove the fish from the oven, flake it and combine with the mashed potato and the parsley. Season well. Let the mixture cool until it can be handled, then mould it into four cakes. Coat the cakes with flour.

Put 1–2 tablespoons of the olive oil in a frying pan over a medium heat, add the fish cakes and fry for 4–5 minutes each side, until golden.

For the sauce, put the yoghurt, lemon zest and capers in a small bowl. Mix in the coriander and salt and pepper, ready to serve with the fish cakes.

For the salad, put the mixed salad leaves in a serving dish, mix in the fennel and drizzle with olive oil and balsamic vinegar. Serve the fish cakes with a squeeze of lemon.

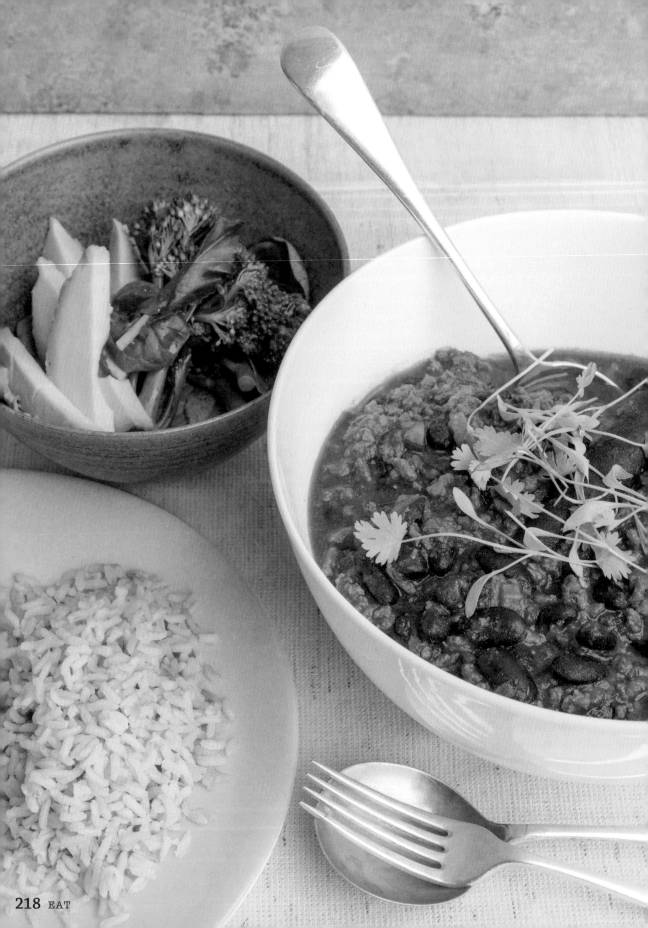

chilli con carne

This old family favourite is the ultimate warming
meal. As it stores well in the fridge or freezer,
it's the perfect dish to whip out when everyone
is ravenous after an active day!

1–2 tablespoons olive oil
1 small onion, diced
2 garlic cloves, crushed
1 celery stick, diced
1 carrot, peeled
2 sticks of cinnamon
1 teaspoon ground cumin
500 g/1 lb minced beef
150 g/5 oz mushrooms diced
1 tin of chopped tomatoes
2 tablespoons tomato puree
600ml/1 pint chicken stock
400 g/14 oz kidney beans
2 teaspoons Worcestershire sauce
1 teaspoon chilli flakes (optional)
Salt and pepper
Brown rice, coriander and a side
order of broccoli or avocado, to serve

SERVES 4-6

Heat the olive oil in a saucepan over a medium–high
heat. Add the onion, garlic, celery, whole carrot,
cinnamon and cumin and cook for a few minutes
until softened.

Add the minced beef, stirring until all the mince has
turned brown. Add the mushrooms, tinned tomatoes,
tomato puree and chicken stock. Simmer for 20–25
minutes. Give it the occasional stir as it cooks and
season well.

Add the kidney beans. Worcestershire sauce, chilli flakes
(if using) and cook for a further 20–25 minutes. Remove
the carrot and cinnamon sticks.

Serve with brown rice, coriander and a side order
of broccoli or avocado.

TIP – *If you're not a meat eater, you could substitute
the minced beef with a variety of beans, such as
pinto beans, black beans, lentils or chickpeas
(240 g/8 oz in total weight).*

prawn skewers with squash and courgette ribbons

These prawn skewers can be cooked on the hob or on a hot barbecue. It's worth investing in a spiralizer to make the vegetable ribbons.

200–300 g/7–10½ oz raw king prawns
2 garlic cloves, crushed
Zest of 1 lemon
5 tablespoons olive oil
12–15 cherry tomatoes
150 g/5 oz courgette
150 g/5 oz butternut squash, peeled and cut into chunks
Salt and black pepper
Parsley, to garnish
Chicory leaves to serve (optional)

SERVES 2 (2 SKEWERS EACH)

TIP - *If you don't have a spiralizer, use a vegetable peeler to peel the courgette and squash into thin strips.*

In a bowl, combine the prawns with half of the garlic, lemon zest, 1–2 tablespoons of olive oil, and salt and pepper. Leave to marinate for 20 minutes.

Thread 3–4 prawns onto a skewer. Place the skewers in the fridge until you're ready to cook them.

Heat 1 tablespoon of oil in a medium-sized pan over a medium heat. Add the rest of the garlic and cherry tomatoes and cook for 2–3 minutes until the tomatoes have softened and some juices have come out. Take off the heat and set aside.

Using a spiralizer, make the vegetable spaghetti by feeding the courgette and squash through the device. Put the tomatoes back on a medium heat, add the vegetable spaghetti and cook for a further 5–8 minutes, gently stirring. Turn off the heat and set aside.

Heat 1 tablespoon of oil in a frying pan over a high heat or on a hot barbecue. Add the prawn skewers and cook for 6 minutes, or until the prawns are a vibrant pink colour. Serve with chicory leaves (optional) and sprinkle on chopped parsley.

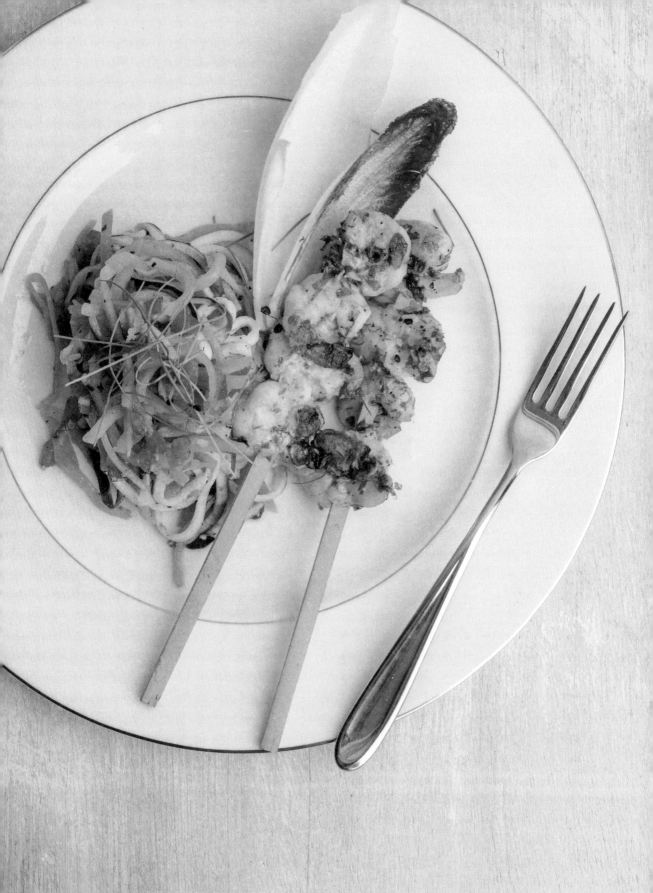

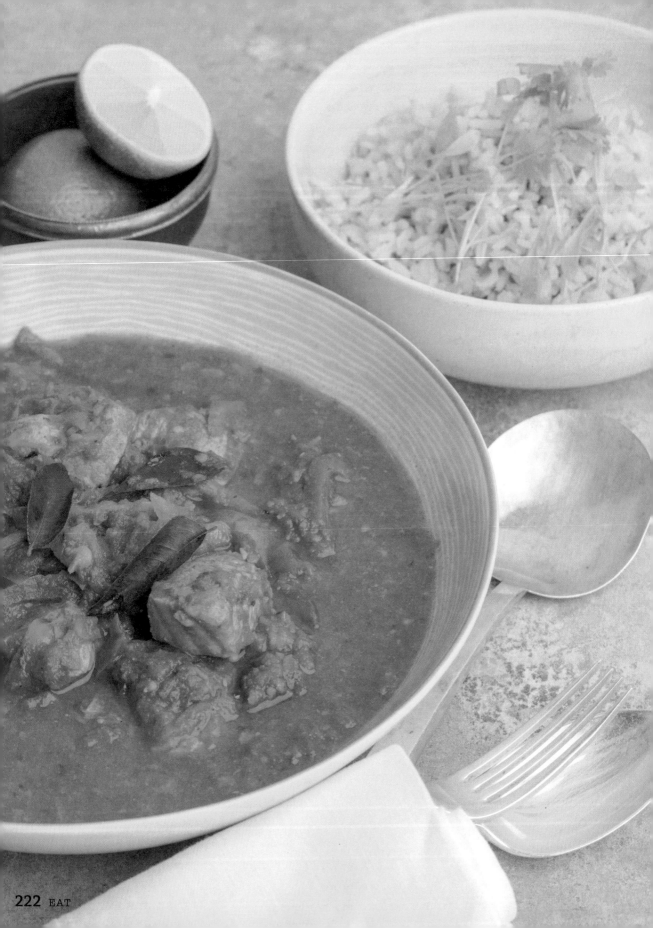

chicken curry

This is a real family favourite, a meal that makes
a regular appearance in the Terry household!
Served with rice, it's gluten-free too.

2 teaspoons ground coriander
1 teaspoon ground cumin
1 teaspoon black pepper
1 teaspoon turmeric
Pinch of paprika
3 tablespoons tikka masala paste
4 skinless chicken breasts, diced
into chunks
60 g/2 oz fresh ginger
4 tablespoons vegetable oil
2 medium onions, finely sliced
4 garlic cloves, finely sliced
4 tomatoes
1 tin of chopped tomatoes
6–8 curry leaves
1 green pepper, deseeded
and thinly sliced
Salt and black pepper
Brown rice, coriander, lime and
yoghurt (optional), to serve

SERVES 4

In a small bowl, mix up the ground coriander, cumin, black pepper, turmeric, paprika and tikka masala paste. Rub half of this mix into the diced chicken breast and leave for an hour in the fridge.

Peel the fresh ginger and grate finely. In a large frying pan with a lid, heat 2 tablespoons of the vegetable oil. Add the onion, garlic and ginger and cook until it is softened and has a little colour. Add the other half of the spice mix and cook for a further 10–12 minutes. Set aside.

Heat the remaining oil in another frying pan, then add the diced and marinated chicken and fry for around 5–6 minutes. Set aside.

Prick the skin of the 4 fresh tomatoes and then plunge them in boiling water for 15 seconds. Remove, leave to cool and peel them. Roughly chop the tomatoes and add to the frying pan containing the onion along with the tin of tomatoes, the curry leaves and 375 ml/1½ cups of water, salt and pepper. Cook on a low heat for 20–25 minutes. Add the chicken, finely sliced green pepper and cook for a further 20 minutes.

Serve with brown rice, coriander leaves, a twist of lime and a tablespoon of yoghurt (optional).

veggie sharing plate

If you have friends or family coming round, serve up this colourful sharing plate of roasted veggies and mozzarella. It's great either on its own or with the fillet steak sharing plate (see overleaf).

1 sweet potato, peeled and cut into chunks
300 g/10½ oz mixed baby peppers, deseeded and cut in half, leaving the stalks on
A few sprigs of thyme
2 courgettes
2 red onions
105 ml/3.7 fl. oz olive oil
4 tablespoons balsamic vinegar
2 garlic cloves, sliced
2 x 125 g mozzarella balls
Half a bag mixed leaves or rocket
Half a bunch of basil
Salt and pepper

SERVES 3-4

Preheat the oven to 180°C/350°F.

Put the sweet potato on a baking tray, sprinkle with salt and pepper, and roast in the oven for 20–25 minutes. Five or ten minutes after you've put the sweet potato in the oven, put the baby peppers on another baking tray, add some of the thyme and a little olive oil and roast in the oven for 12–15 minutes until they soften.

Cut each courgette long ways, into 4–5 slices. Peel and cut the onions in half and then into 8 wedges. Put the courgette and onion in a bowl and combine with 2 tablespoons of the olive oil, 2 tablespoons of the balsamic vinegar, the rest of the thyme, the sliced garlic, salt and pepper. Then cook under a hot grill for 10–15 minutes until the onion and courgette soften and colour.

Arrange the roasted vegetables on a large plate. Tear the mozzarella and place in the middle of the plate, sprinkling it with rocket and basil. In a small bowl, mix 3 tablespoons of olive oil with 2 tablespoons of balsamic vinegar and pour over the veggies.

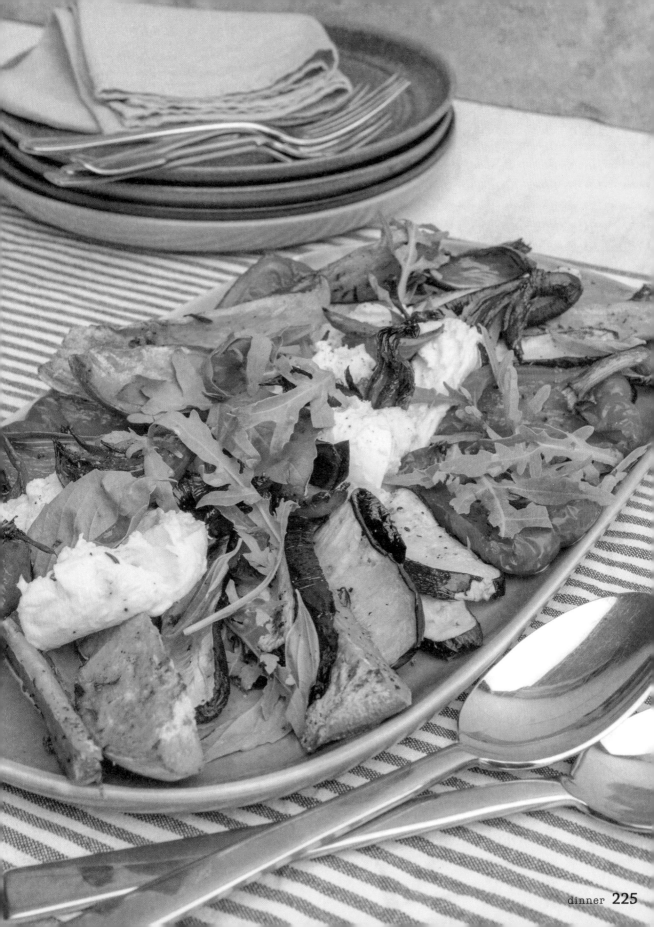

fillet steak sharing plate

Vegetarians, look away! Juicy slices of fillet steak look really appetizing on this sharing plate. This could accompany the veggie sharing plate on the previous page.

800 g/1.7 lbs fillet steak from your butcher (ideally the middle piece so it cooks evenly)
4 sprigs of thyme, leaves picked
4 tablespoons olive oil
1 small broccoli
200 g/7 oz frozen peas
4 tomatoes on the vine, sliced
Handful of rocket or watercress
Ready-made hollandaise sauce
Salt and pepper

SERVES 4

Preheat the oven to 200°C/390°F.

Put a frying pan on the hob and leave for a minute or so to get hot. Season your fillet with salt and pepper, the thyme and the olive oil. Place the steak in the pan and fry over a high heat for 5 minutes, turning it until the meat has a good brown colour all over.

Place the pan in the preheated oven and cook for 10–12 minutes for medium-rare, or to your liking. Remove from the oven and allow it to rest for 15 minutes before slicing.

Bring a pan of water to the boil. Cook the broccoli florets for 2–3 minutes. Put your frozen peas in a sieve and strain the broccoli over them, then toss with salt and pepper. This will be enough cooking time for the peas.

Serve on a large plate or board with tomato, rocket or watercress and hollandaise sauce.

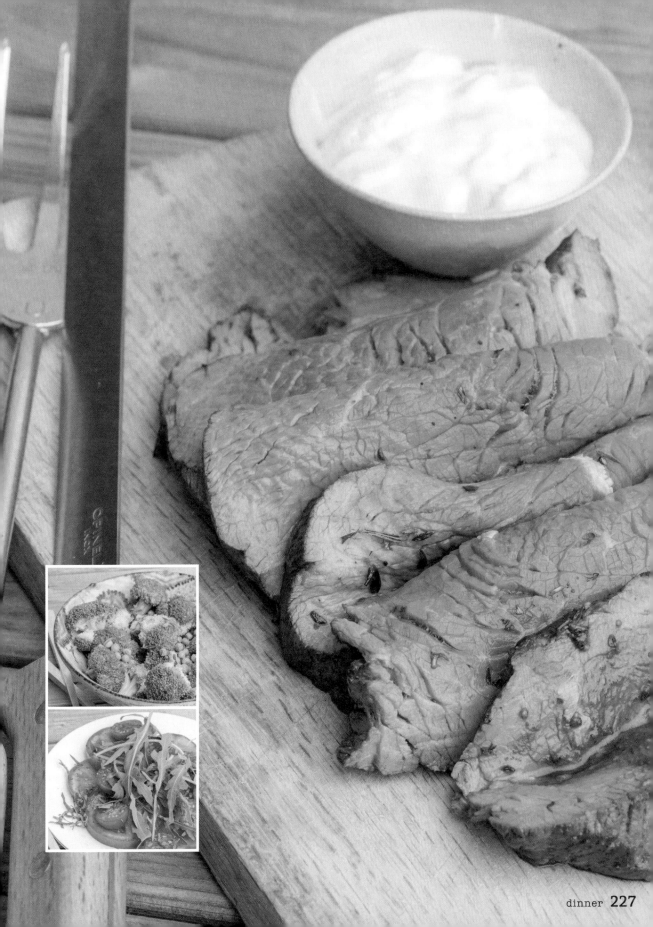

squash and spinach curry

This vegetarian and gluten-free curry is warming but not too spicy. Just add a few more chilli flakes and curry powder if you want to spice things up.

1 butternut squash, peeled and cut into chunks
2 teaspoons ground cumin
2 teaspoons ground coriander
2 teaspoons mild curry powder
Half a teaspoon chilli flakes
1 teaspoon ground ginger
2 garlic cloves, crushed
4 tablespoons vegetable or rapeseed oil
1 tablespoon tomato puree
250 ml/9 fl. oz (or just over half a tin) of good coconut milk
2 handfuls of fresh spinach
Rice, flat bread and yoghurt, to serve
Coriander and limes, to garnish

SERVES 4

Preheat the oven to 180°C/350°F.

Put the squash in a roasting pan, add half the quantity of each of the spices (cumin, coriander, curry powder, chilli flakes, ginger and garlic) with 2 tablespoons of the oil. Mix together and bake for 20 minutes. When cooked, remove the squash from the oven and set aside.

Heat the remaining oil in a large pan over a medium heat. Add the rest of the cumin, coriander, curry powder, chilli flakes, ginger and garlic and cook for 1 minute until you smell a slight aroma. Add the tomato puree, coconut milk, 500 ml/2 cups of water and stir. Simmer for 30 minutes.

Blend the curry mixture either in a liquidizer or hand-held blender until you have a thin but creamy sauce. Return it to the saucepan, add the squash and fresh spinach, and cook for a minute over a low heat to soften the spinach.

Serve with steamed rice, flat bread, yoghurt, coriander and lime halves, and garnish with coriander.

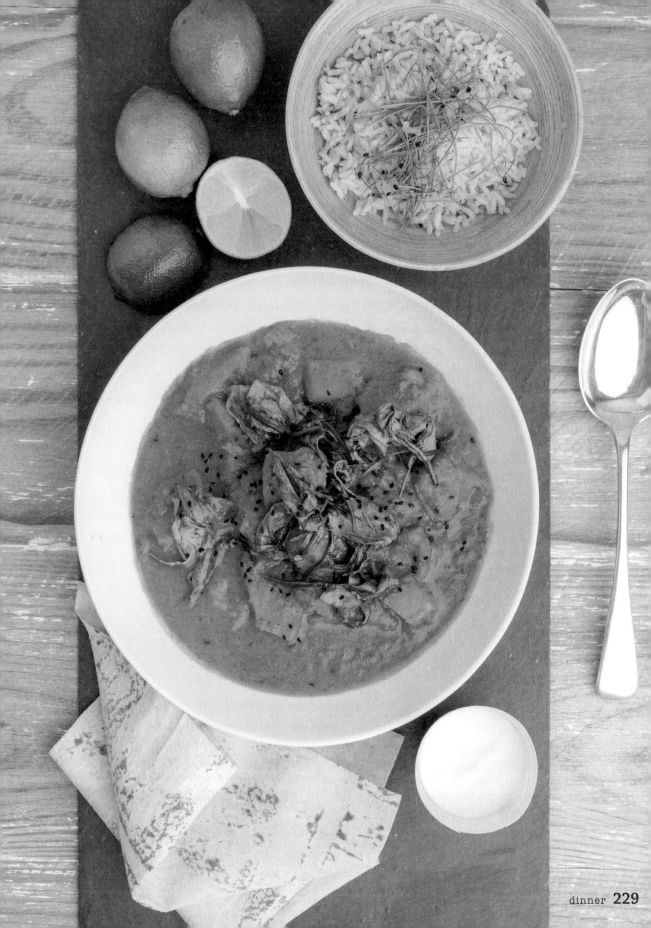

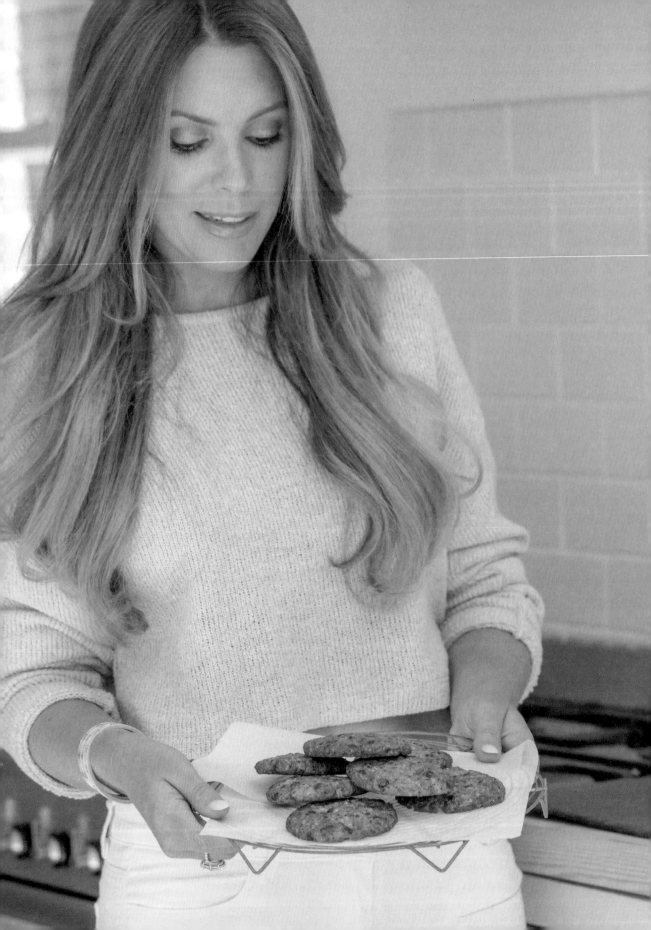

sweet treats

oat, poppy seed and choc chip cookies

These are a healthier alternative to most shop-bought biscuits, containing less sugar and a combination of plain and spelt flour.

60–70 g/2–2 ½ oz spelt flour
60–70 g/2–2 ½ oz plain flour
45 g/1½ oz rolled oats
90 g/3 oz demerara sugar
2 teaspoons poppy seeds
Half a teaspoon bicarbonate of soda
120 g/4 oz butter
1 tablespoon honey
1 egg
100g dark chocolate buttons or bar of chocolate, chopped (preferably 50–70% cocoa)

MAKES 8

TIP – The cookie dough keeps well in the fridge for a week, or you can have the ball of dough in the freezer ready to go.

Preheat the oven to 190°C/375°F.

Put the spelt flour, plain flour, oats, sugar, poppy seeds and bicarbonate of soda in a bowl and mix together.

Add the butter and honey to the bowl and, using a hand-held whisk or blender, mix until it resembles buttery breadcrumbs. Then add the egg and chocolate and stir until it combines into a big ball. (Don't overdo it, use the pulse button if using a blender.)

Put the mixture in a bowl and chill in the fridge for an hour. Line a baking tray with parchment.

When the mixture is chilled, mould it into eight balls. Then put them on the baking tray, pressing down slightly with the heal of your hand or the back of a spoon. Keep some space between them as they spread when cooking. Bake for 12–15 minutes.

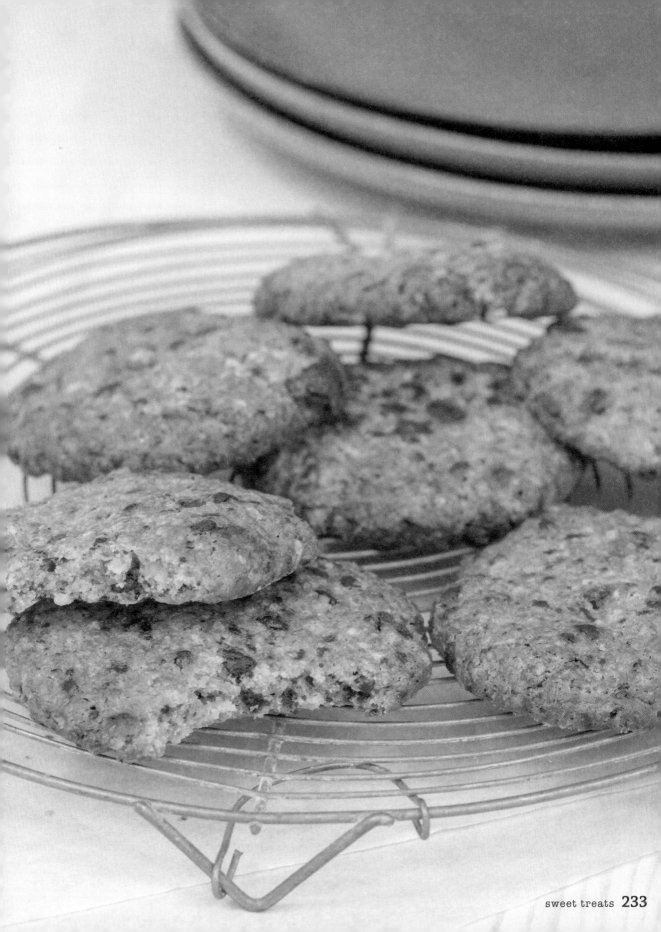

lollies

These are super-healthy lollies with no added sugar. Your children will love them – just don't tell them how healthy they are!

mango lolly

2 ripe mangoes, peeled and destoned
250 ml/8 ½ fl. oz cloudy apple juice
Squeeze of lime
1 tablespoon coconut yoghurt or plain yoghurt

MAKES 4

Blend all the ingredients in a food processor or blender and pour into lolly moulds. Add lolly sticks and freeze overnight. These lollies will keep for a month in the freezer.

berry lolly

180 g/6 oz frozen raspberries and blueberries
2 teaspoons honey
250 ml/8 ½ fl. oz cloudy apple juice

MAKES 4

Put the berries in a saucepan, add the honey and cook over a low heat for 5 minutes, stirring once or twice. Take off the heat and add the apple juice. If you would prefer not to have the seeds, push the mixture through a sieve before pouring into the moulds. Freeze overnight. These lollies will keep for a month in the freezer.

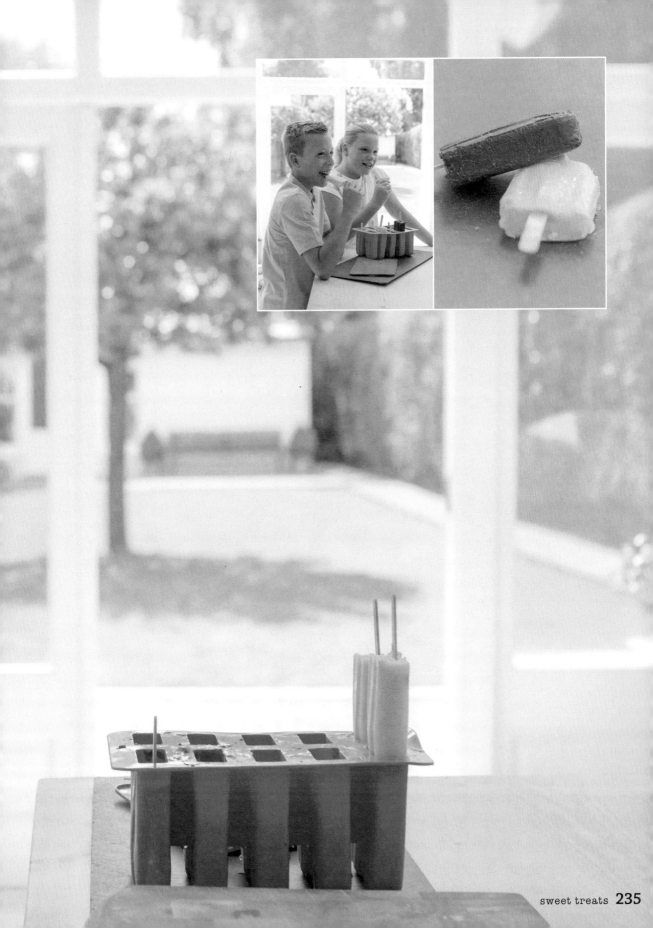

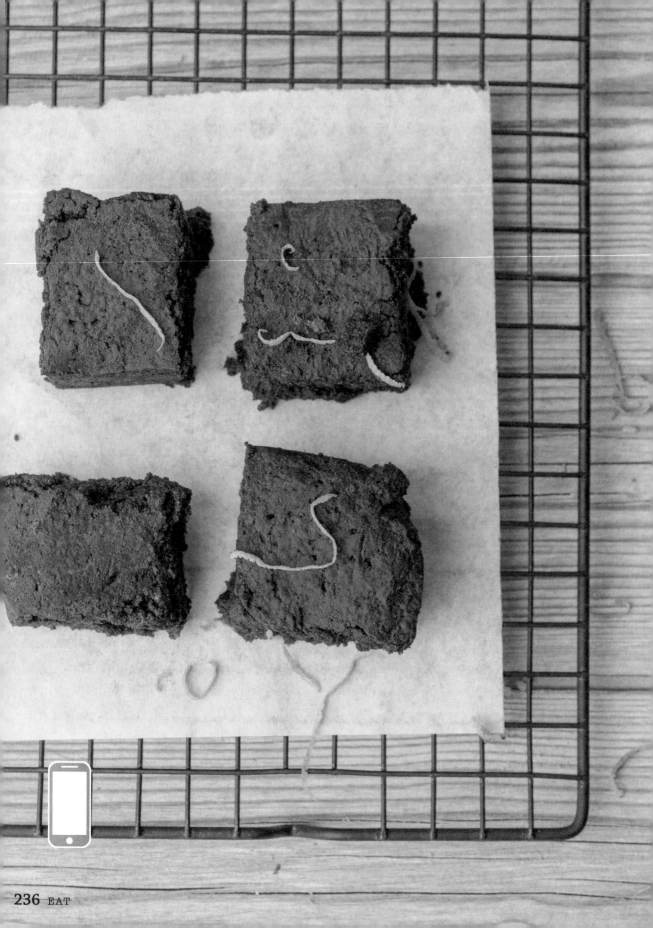

chocolate, coconut and orange brownies

These brownies are beautifully rich and gooey and really satisfy those chocolate cravings. They're made with coconut flour, which is a healthy, gluten-free alternative to other wheat-based flours.

250 g/9 oz dark chocolate (preferably 50% cocoa)
100 ml/3 ½ fl. oz coconut oil
180 g/6 oz honey
150 g/5 oz brown sugar
5 eggs
50 g/2 oz coconut flour
Zest of 1 orange
1 teaspoon gluten-free or regular baking powder
50 g/2 oz ground almonds
40 g/1½ oz cocoa powder

MAKES 10-12

Preheat the oven to 180°C/350°F. Line a 30-cm/12-inch square baking tray with parchment paper (ensuring you line the sides as well).

Put the chocolate and coconut oil in a heatproof bowl and place over a saucepan of simmering water until it melts.

Using either a hand-held electric whisk or food mixer, whisk the honey, sugar and eggs for 5 minutes until thick and creamy in consistency.

Add the melted chocolate to the egg mix. Whisk in, just for a few seconds, the coconut flour, orange zest, baking powder, ground almonds and cocoa powder. Then, using a spoon, give the mix a gentle stir, checking everything is fully combined at the bottom of the bowl.

Pour into the lined baking tray and bake for 30 minutes. The mixture will be soft to touch but will firm up when it cools. Remove from the oven and leave to cool before slicing.

frozen yoghurt with berries

A refreshing and healthy dessert that will
please friends and family. The berries add
a great splash of colour.

400 g/14 oz whole milk strained
Greek yoghurt
4 tablespoons mild honey
Zest of 1 lime
Juice of half a lemon
Half a vanilla pod or 1 teaspoon of
vanilla essence
Fresh berries, to serve

Put the yoghurt in the freezer for 20 minutes to chill.

Remove the yoghurt from the freezer and place in a bowl
with the honey, lime zest and lemon juice. Whisk with a
hand-held electric whisk or put in a food processor until
smooth. If using a vanilla pod, cut it in half lengthwise,
then use the back of small knife to scrape out the seeds
of one half. Mix the seeds or vanilla essence into the
yoghurt. Scrape the mixture into a medium-sized plastic
container with a lid. Chill in the freezer for 30–40 minutes.

Serve with fresh berries of your choice.

TIP – *This frozen yoghurt is meant to be eaten after
a short time in the freezer. If frozen for a long period
of time, it will get very hard. If that happens, simply
leave it out at room temperature for 15 minutes to
soften before scooping.*

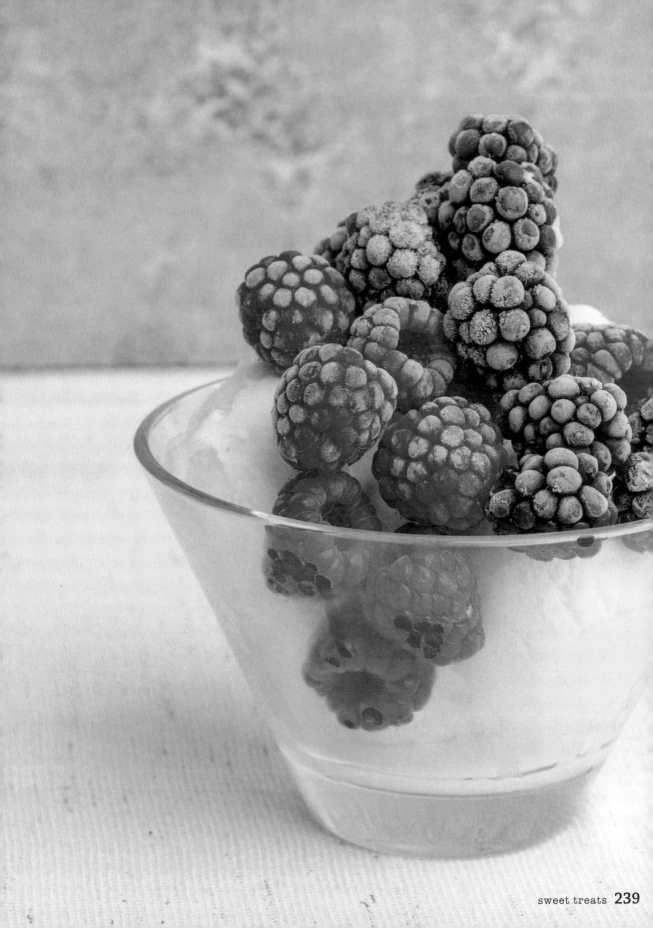

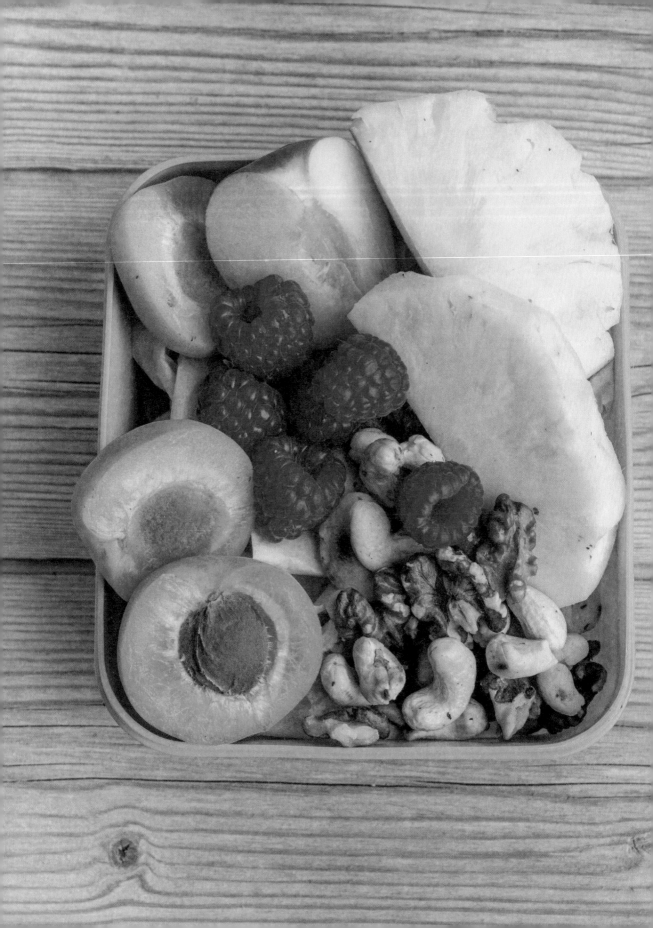

snacks

protein balls

I promise you, these snacks are absolutely delicious. They include the perfect combination of protein, carbs and fats and provide a real energy boost when you've had an active day. If you don't have time to make them, you can also buy ready-made ones from nutri-bombz.com

50 g–60 g/1½ –2 oz flaxseed, sunflower and pumpkin seed mix, (or just pumpkin and sunflower seeds if the flaxseed is not available)
40 g/1½ oz cashews
225 g/8 oz dried dates
Zest of 1 orange
Half a teaspoon fennel seeds
2 tablespoons chunky peanut butter
1 tablespoon tahini
30 g/1 oz rolled oats

MAKES AROUND 10 BALLS

TIP - *If you put these protein balls in an airtight container, they will keep in the fridge for 10 days. They can also be frozen without the seeds on.*

Put the seeds and cashews in a small frying pan and toast them over a low heat for a few minutes until they turn a golden colour. Put to one side.

Put the dates in a saucepan, cover with water and bring to the boil. Then take off the heat and leave to stand for around 20 minutes; they just need to be a little soft to make the balls.

Put the toasted cashews, orange zest and fennel seeds in a blender. Give the blender a small pulse to break up the cashews slightly. Then add in the softened dates, peanut butter and tahini, and blitz. The mixture should come together in one ball.

Take the mixture out of the blender and put it in a bowl. Add the oats and roughly combine them by hand. Put the mixture in the fridge for 1–2 hours until it is chilled and more manageable.

Mould into 3 cm/1 inch round balls. Roll in the toasted seeds and put back into the fridge for a further 30 minutes.

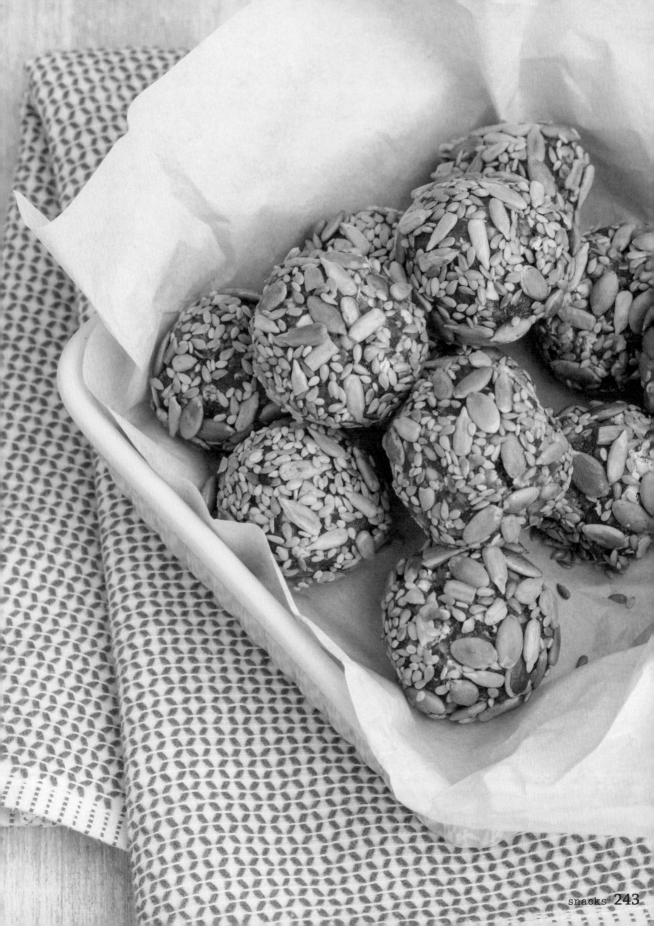

beetroot and hummus dips

These dips make fantastic, kid-friendly snacks or lunchtime treats. Served with lots of colourful vegetables, they're also great at parties or get-togethers with friends.

beetroot

SERVES 3-4

250–300 g/9–10½ oz cooked beetroot
3–4 tablespoons olive oil
2–3 tablespoons Cabernet Sauvignon vinegar or good balsamic vinegar
Salt and black pepper

Put all the ingredients in a blender, season and blitz until everything is nice and smooth.

hummus

SERVES 3-4

1 400 g/14 oz tin of chickpeas
2 heaped tablespoons tahini
2 garlic cloves
Zest and juice of 1 large lemon
3–4 tablespoons olive oil, plus extra for serving
Salt and black pepper

Put all the ingredients in a blender, add 125 ml/4 fl. oz water and blitz until you get a smooth consistency. Serve in a dipping bowl with a little extra olive oil on top.

TIP - You can serve both dips with carrot sticks, thinly sliced cucumber, baby peppers, cooked tender stem broccoli, cauliflower, radishes, gem leaves, flat bread – or any vegetable or accompaniment of your choice! Both dips freeze really well so you can always make more than you need and keep any leftovers in the freezer.

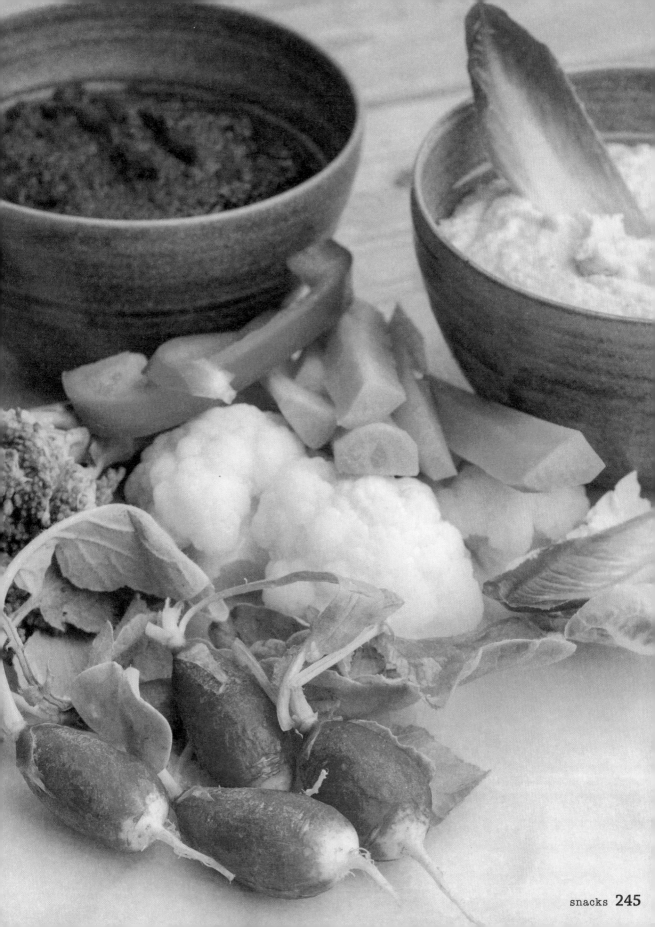

fruits, nuts and seeds

Fruits and berries, nuts and seeds make super-healthy snacks to keep you and your family going through the day. I'll often have nuts and seeds to hand as they are an excellent source of protein and good fats, while fruits and berries provide healthy vitamins and nutrients.

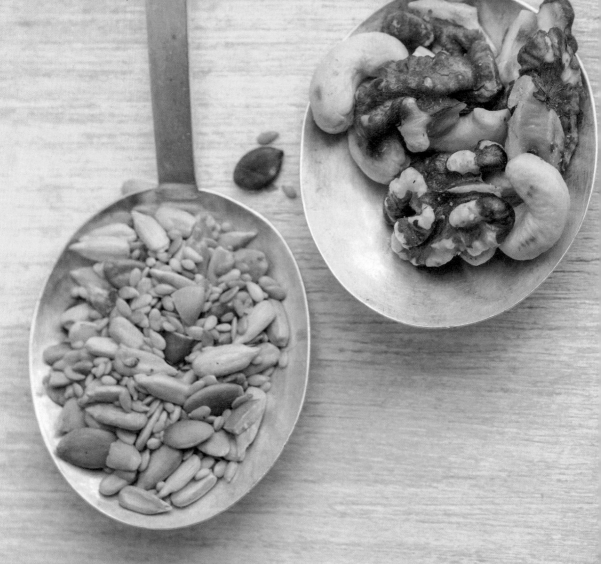

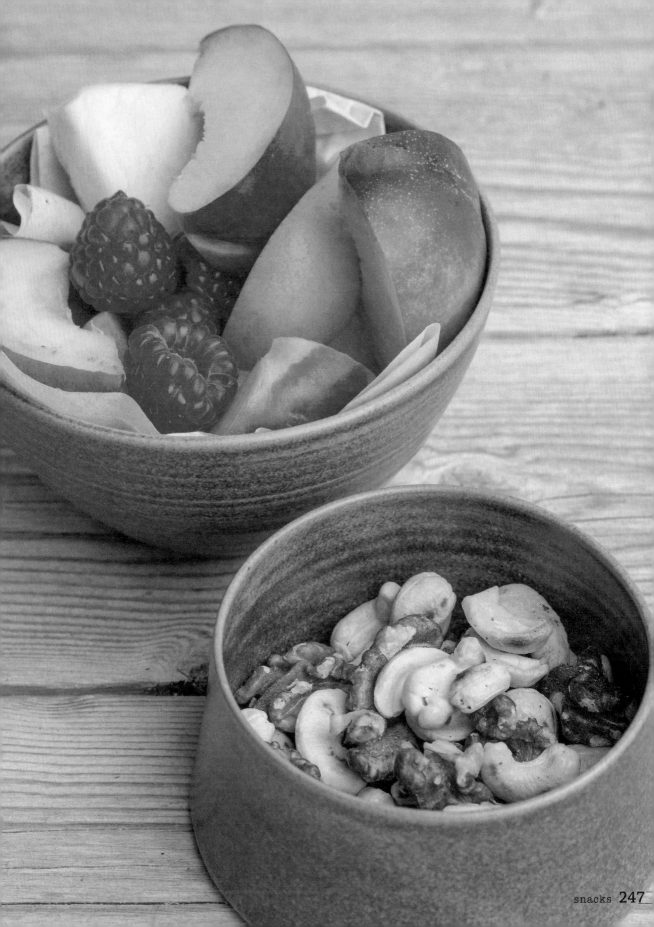

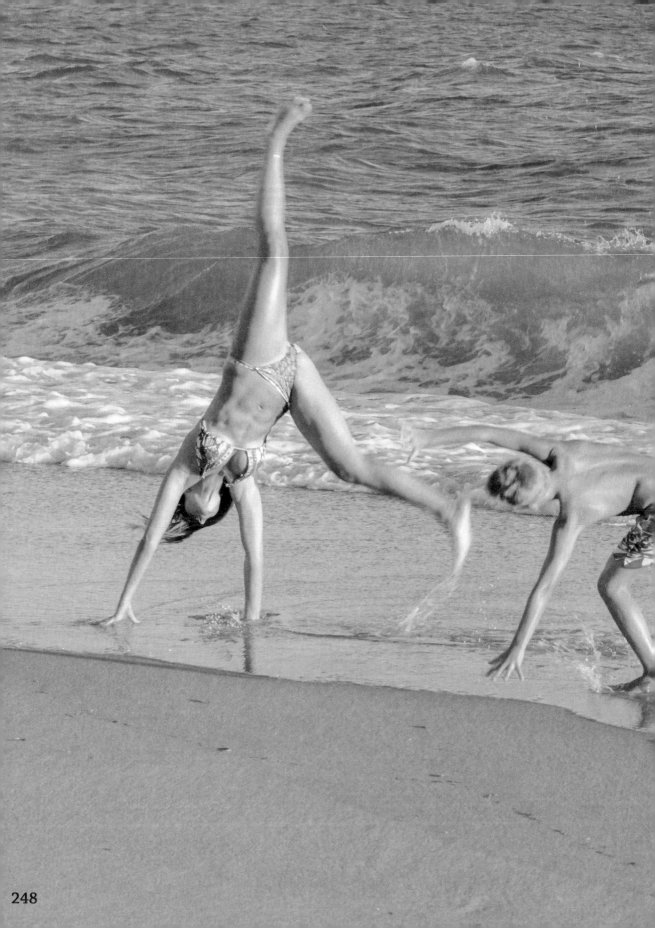

Enjoy the journey!

So now you've got some of my favourite recipes, the low-down on my workout programme and some realistic tips on how to get going, keep motivated and ultimately achieve that strong and healthy body you've always wanted. I won't pretend this is easy – it's a long journey and you have to work hard, eat well and stay committed.

What's helped to keep me on track are my friends and family. So try working out with your buddies, encourage each other, try new things and have a good time in the process! I'd love to hear about your buddy workout stories so why not share them on my instagram page @toniterry26

I wish you every success in your journey – here's to a happier, healthier you.

Toni Terry x

Index

Acknowledgements

Thanks to

John: I wouldn't have gone through with the book if it wasn't for you, hubby. You believed in me and supported, encouraged and pushed me as you always do. Thank you for giving me the confidence and the courage to do this. I will be forever grateful. I love you, Mr T. Georgie and Summer: my two beautiful children. You have been so supportive and helpful for mummy. Thank you for all your help in the photo shoots – you kept me smiling and giggling even when I was nervous! I love you both. Mum and Dad: for always being there for me. You have believed in me all my life. No matter how big or small my dreams and ambitions, you have encouraged and supported me every step of the way. I love you both very much.

Claire: for being part of my book – it means so much to me. Even though I know you hate having your picture taken, you were there supporting me and making everyone laugh. You're a very special friend and I'm so grateful for all the time and effort that you put in to help make this book. Connie: for being part of my book. You have been so supportive and we have had so much fun and laughs along the way. You're a true inspiration not only as a friend but to many women out there. Bradley: for all your help and support with my book – your knowledge has been invaluable. You have helped me to achieve the body I always wanted and pushed us girls to our limits week in week out!

Emma: for being there for me throughout this whole experience of writing a book. You have gone over and above for me and I'm truly grateful. I look forward to working with you on many more projects. Michael: for showing me how to relax in front of the lens! You helped me so much with your kind but professional way. I'm so thrilled with the pictures and look forward to working with you again. Natalie: for helping me through such a fantastic experience and for all your help, support and tips. It's been a pleasure working with you. Richard: to you and Leigh for coming to me and believing in me to do such an amazing project. I have loved every minute and look forward to the next project!

FURTHER ONLINE INFO

There are loads of apps and online sources and communities out there that will help you on your fitness and health journey.

BUDDIES

If you're on the lookout for like-minded people to work out with, why not try:

Buddyup.com – finds individuals or groups that you can hook up with for various sports and activities.

Findafitnessbuddy.co.uk – tracks down workout buddies that share your fitness goals, love your sports and are a similar fitness level to you.

Meetup.com – find all sorts of groups, from running groups and general fitness clubs to salsa and ping pong!

KEEPING TRACK

Myfitnesspal.com – helps you to keep track of what you're eating and the activity you do, and provides support and tips via its online community.

TIMERS

Here are some mobile apps that will help you time your HIIT and circuit workouts.

Interval Timer: Timing for HIIT Training, Workouts
Interval Training Assistant
Circuit Training Timer
Bit Timer
Seconds – Interval Timer
iSmooth Run

GENERAL

Also check out my Instagram page @ToniTerry26 for workout videos, shots of me and the family, buddy workout stories and much more!

Find out more about trainer Bradley Simmonds on bradleysimmonds.co.uk

More info and pictures of my workout buddy Connie Simmonds can be found on her Instagram page @cbeauty_

Delicious, ready-made protein balls can be purchased from nutri-bombz.com

Published by Lagom in 2017
Lagom is an imprint of
Kings Road Publishing,
3.08, The Plaza,
535 Kings Road,
Chelsea Harbour,
London, SW10 0SZ

A CIP catalogue of this book is available from the British Library.

Project edited and managed by Emma Marriott/Tall Tree Ltd

Photography by Michael Wicks, except for: pages 16, 19, 21, 22, 24 supplied by John and Toni Terry; 23 photographer Andy Hooper/ REX/SHUTTERSTOCK; 61 top middle by LightField Shudios/ Shutterstock

Design by Paul at paultilby.com

Recipes devised and tested by Janie Fraser at bakedsalt.co. uk. All recipes have been tested and follow general nutritional guidelines

Food photography styled by Michael Wicks, Emma Marriott and Janie Fraser

Hair and make-up by Kim Douglas, Sarah Tyrell and Sina Velke/CLM (London)

Swimwear provided for John and Georgie Terry by Thomas Royall

Printed and bound by Rotolito Lombarda, Italy

ISBN 978-1-91160-052-7

Copyright © Toni Terry, 2017